FiT-KiDS...

GETTING KIDS 'HOOKED' ON FITNESS FUN!

BY

MANDY LADERER

1ST EDITION
ALLURE PUBLISHING

"FIT-KIDS"...Getting Kids Hooked On Fitness Fun!

Published by ALLURE PUBLISHING
1470 Old Country Road, Suite 320, Plainview, NY 11803

Library Of Congress Cataloging in Publication Data
Library Of Congress Catalog Card Number: 93-74028

ISBN: 0-9639178-1-1

Printed in the United States of America

To my husband, Michael,

my daughters, Alissa & Ashley,

Mom & Dad,

and my brothers, Colin & Terry.

Acknowledgement

Writing this book has been most challenging, exciting and rewarding. As always, a project of this kind can never be accomplished by only one person.

My deepest thanks go to Larry and Gerry Parish for the long hours they spent assisting me with formatting and editing my manuscript. I appreciate their complete belief in my book as well as their practical advice and persistant encouragement.

Thanks to photographer, Tom Sammut who spent many hours in the cold temperatures in order to produce the photographs used in this book.

Thanks to my husband, Michael, who has been patient with me throughout the years and for helping me reach for my dreams.

Thanks to my mother for her guidance with her years of experience with children.

Thanks to my father who encouraged me to write at an early age.

I would like to thank all of the wonderful "FIT-KIDS" I have had the pleasure to work with through the years.

I would like to extend a special thanks to Lisa and Jenna who spent many long hours posing for the photographs featured in the book.

Extra special thanks to my daughter, Alissa. In addition to posing for the photographs as well, Alissa inspired me to work with children the day she was born.

And thanks to you, the reader.

"FIT-KIDS"...
Getting Your Child Hooked On Fitness Fun!

TABLE OF CONTENTS

FIT-KIDS: GETTING KIDS "HOOKED" ON FITNESS FUN!

CHAPTER 1

CAUTION; CHILDREN NOT AT PLAY!

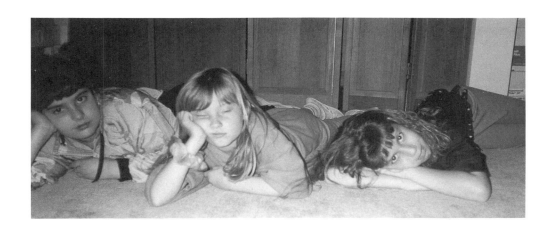

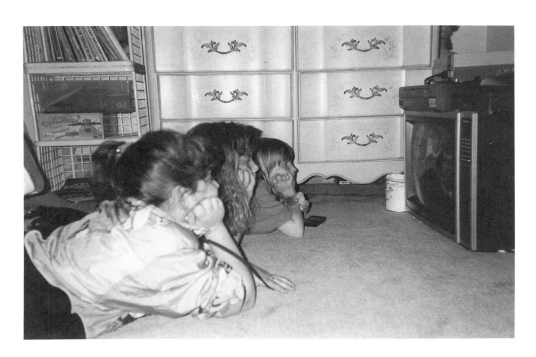

One

Millions of children face the prospect of serious diseases and decreased life span because of sedentary lifestyles and poor nutrition habits. Presently, children as young as six years of age weigh more and have considerably more body fat than twenty years ago.

Only thirty-two percent of children between the ages of six to seventeen meet the minimum requirements of cardiovascular fitness, flexibility, and upper strength.

Approximately forty percent of children between the ages of five to eight have at least one heart disease risk factor. According to The Presidents Council Of Physical Fitness, several heart disease risk factors have been identified as physical inactivity, obesity, high cholesterol, and high blood pressure.

It is the natural inclination of a child to be active, but parents should be aware of various influences that may inhibit him or her on a daily basis. An average American child watches three to seven hours of television (including video games) and is a passenger in a moving vehicle for at least ten to fifteen miles every day. As a result, children are sitting for an extended period of time (an average of three to seven hours). While eight hours a day must be used for sleep, this leaves very little time allowed for physical activities.

Children develop television habits at a very young age. Parents tend to use television as an instant babysitter. Unfortunately, this type of behavior detracts from exercise for children and adults alike. Moreover, the lack of exercise experienced consistently will reinforce the practice of watching television instead of engaging in some type of activity. While the regimen of watching television may rob the body of essential cardiovascular maintenance, the problem becomes compounded when unhealthy snacks are consumed as part of the ritual.

As counter-productive as television viewing can be, playing video games can sometimes be worse. As the child is still sitting in front of the television, he or she may become fixated with a particular game. There is always another level of challenge introduced, and therefore the amount of time spent sitting in the same position increases.

An example should be set for children by introducing television viewing and video game playing limitations. However, this should not be done as a form of punishment. Instead, the time usually spent in front of the television can be substituted with many fun and healthy activities. The following chapters in this book will introduce several approaches to get children (and adults) away from the television.

The amount of of which people walk has greatly decreased with the use of cars and public transportation such as buses and trains. Presently, the average person will exert as little physical activity as possible to get to their destination. How many times have you witnessed a person drive around a parking lot several times in order to find the closest parking space to a store? It's no wonder that most children want to be driven all over the place instead of walking or biking. The children are following the examples which have been made by their parents.

Modern conveniences such as drive-up telephone booths, drive-through supermarkets, fast food restaurants, and banks have contributed to a decrease of physical activity. It has become necessary to perhaps re-evaluate the way our lives shape the future lifestyles of children. Although sometimes difficult, parents may choose to walk up to a telephone booth or into a market, restaurant, or bank. After only a couple of times of practicing this behavior, it is probable that many errands performed with children can be converted to become fun and rewarding exercise excursions.

When children are young and are in preschool, they are allowed a certain amount of free expression which is manifested in activities. As children move up in grades, the amount of mobility and exploration becomes limited. Out of the average six hour school day, approximately five hours of this time is spent sitting behind a desk.

The structure of many physical education classes do not properly utilize time to maximize the amount of activity a child experiences. Children may spend an extended amount of time waiting in line for their turn to "play". It is important for parents to become involved with the school that their child attends for many reasons. The physical fitness program of a school should be a primary concern as well.

Just because children attend Physical Education classes, it doesn't necessarily mean they're getting physical. A survey of fifth grade Physical Education classes in Texas schools found students to be moderately to vigorously active during less than nine percent of class time. The amount of time children engaged in physical activity added up to approximately ten minute per week.

The reason for the extremely low ratio was because much of the time, students watch or await their turn to play states a study in the AMERICAN JOURNAL OF PUBLIC HEALTH. If instructors were to focus on lifetime activities (ie; jogging, calisthenics, and jumping rope), students could be active fifty percent of the time or more the study concluded.

There are no federal laws mandating physical education. Each state decides if, and how much physical education is required. In 1987, THE ALLIANCE released the results of a study of state physical education requirements called The Shape Of The Nation. This particular study detailed just how much (or how little) physical education is required by the various states. The following excerpts highlight the key areas of the study;

- Only four states require students to take a specific amount of physical education for children in kindergarten through the twelfth grade.
- Illinois is the only state requiring all students from kindergarten through the twelfth grade to attend physical education.
- Only five states require elementary school students to attend physical education thirty minutes per days, five days per week.
- Only five states require high school students to attend Physical Education classes.

The 1992 results of The Shape Of The Nation survey illustrates the following changes which occurred since the 1987 report was issued;

- Six states now require elementary school students to attend Physical Education classes.
- Eight states now require high school students to attend Physical Education classes.

FIT-KIDS: GETTING KIDS "HOOKED" ON FITNESS FUN!

CHAPTER 2

WHY CHILDREN NEED PHYSICAL ACTIVITY

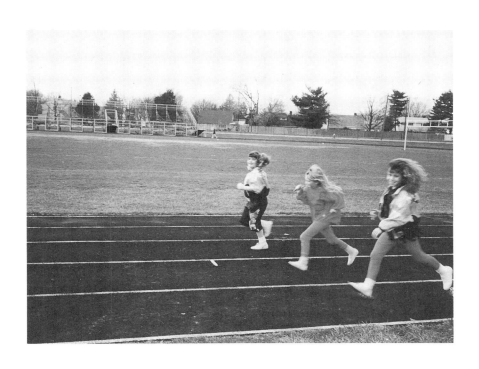

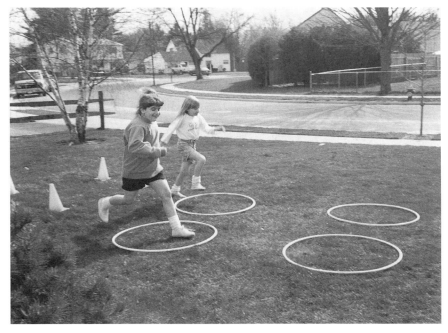

Two

Children require basic guidelines that will lead to a healthy and productive life as adults. Parents and teachers instill sufficient math and reading skills. However, proper exercise instruction is often neglected. Physical activity should become as much of a daily lesson as arithmetic and reading.

Regular physical activity should begin as early as infancy. At this early stage, exercise can become a natural part of a daily routine. Research shows that exercise helps children to develop physically, mentally, and emotionally. Moreover, children that exercise at an early age become more alert, confident, and socially aware.

Good minds thrive in good bodies. Additionally, the ability of a child to learn will increase with physical fitness. Basically, a weak body will become fatigued easily resulting in a decreased ability to concentrate.

Being "out of shape" is associated with a greater chance of scholastic underachievement. The connection between physical fitness and academic accomplishments may be the fact that young people that exercise feel better about themselves. The increased level of self-esteem is reflected onto the study habits.

Exercising on a regular basis will help children improve their motor skills (movement), cognitive skills (thinking), perceptual skills (sensory), balance, and coordination.

A question often raised is "Do fat children grow up to be fat adults?". The answer is that all overweight children do not become obese adults, however, most do. More often than not, the marginally overweight child will grow up to become a "fat" adult.

The dangers of adult obesity are well known. The heavy adult is at a higher risk to develop heart disease or suffer a stroke. In addition, certain forms of cancer have become apparent from not maintaining a healthy diet. This is why it is extremely important to raise a child with a healthy, acceptable weight. The dangers of child obesity have become a large concern today.

Childhood obesity is unhealthy on all accords. There is a definite association between overweight children, elevated blood cholesterol levels, and high blood pressure.

Most overweight children are discriminated against by their peers in school as early as kindergarten. If a child grows up with a negative attitude concerning their own body, he or she will experience a dramatic decrease of self esteem and self confidence.

The child which constantly engages in over eating without participating in an exercise program will become flabby and clumsy. As a result, the child will suffer from fatigue. This in turn, will subsequently lead to a feeling of alienation.

Parents do not have control over the height of their child. However, there are some elements which can be monitored and altered if necessary. By helping children maintain an active lifestyle and eating healthy, various concerns mentioned in this chapter will become nonexistent.

Young people respond well to physical training and can make significant improvements in cardiovascular endurance, body composition, muscular strength, and flexibility. However, children should not be viewed as miniature adults. Rather, their physiologic and psychological differences should be understood, and carefully taken into consideration when implementing any physical training program.

FIT-KIDS: GETTING KIDS "HOOKED" ON FITNESS FUN!

CHAPTER 3
EXERCISE PLAY-DO'S

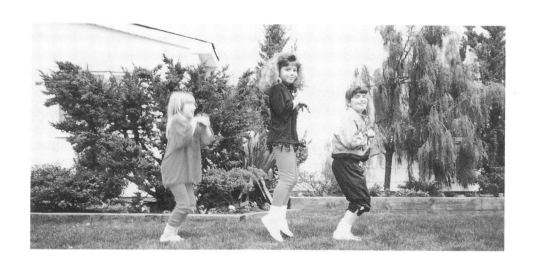

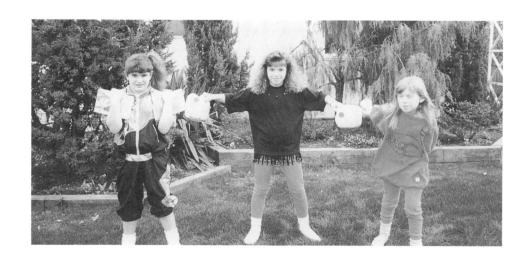

Three

When planning fitness fun for children, it's important to instill a feeling of success. This can be accomplished simply by making sure that all activities are based on a completely noncompetitive philosophy. Additionally, by following the guidelines detailed in this chapter, children can enjoy a variety of aspects that accompany fitness fun.

- Make It Fun:

  If fun is emphasized, fitness will follow. Forcing children to exercise in order to improve their health will never have a long-lasting effect. On the contrary, children may even develop a strong disregard for fitness altogether if a clinical approach is adopted. Moreover, exercise should never be used as a form of punishment.

- Keep Them Moving:

  The attention span of children is limited. It is essential to select a variety of activities, and to keep the kids moving from one to the next. Variety is the spice of life.

- Regularity:

  Incorporating some form of physical activity with a child on a daily basis will help turn exercise into a regular routine similar to brushing teeth.

- Encouragement:

  Support and encourage a child for every accomplishment that is achieved. Focus on the positive. Children will continue to increase their aptitude and endurance when praise is given.

- Music:

  It is a fact that children become uninhibited to move when music is played. That is why it is extremely important to use favorite music of a child when exercising.

- Props:

  Excitement can easily be added to any activity by incorporating props such as scarves, towels, balls, or balloons as an example.

- Participation:

  Nothing motivates a child more than when a parent, adult friend, or teacher participates in a activity together with children.

- Taking One Day At A Time:

  A child should begin slowly, and graduate toward a variety of activities while increasing stamina and strength. A journal or chart can be maintained to track the progress of the child (or children). When a child has visually witnessed their own accomplishments, he or she will become motivated to strive toward higher goals (the Wall Chart Of Success is outlined in chapter seven).

- Reward System:

   Offering a ribbon or small trophy will assist in reinforcing motivation to a child. After an accomplishment of exercise, a reward of this type can be used quite effectively as a tool for motivation. Rewards may be presented daily, weekly, or monthly (rewards are outlined in chapter nine).

- Role models:

   Children learn by example. Parents and teachers must set proper examples when a child is still young and very impressionable. With proper guidance, a child can be lead down the road to fun exercise and healthy eating. A closer look at role models are seen throughout chapter ten.

Many parents and teachers do not realize how important it is to help instill proper exercise and eating habits in children. The earlier in life these health patterns become established, the more likely they will continue throughout one's entire life.

There seems to be a general assumption among adults. Just because children are basically active, they require little or no guidance. However, youngsters need direction and encouragement to achieve their maximum fitness and nutrition potential.

KID'S + YOU = Fun, Effective Kid's Fitness Program

FIT-KIDS: GETTING KIDS "HOOKED" ON FITNESS FUN!

CHAPTER 4
IMAGINATIVE EXERCISE IDEAS FOR KIDS FITNESS

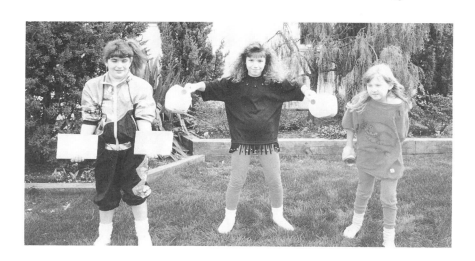

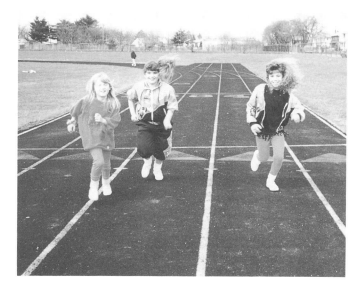

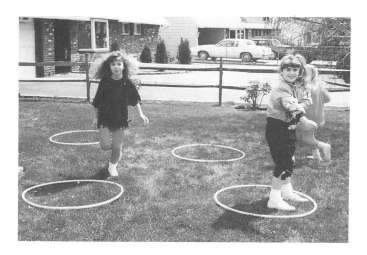

Four

To get kids "hooked on fitness", we must show them how to put spice into traditional aerobics and calisthenics. This can easily be achieved by creating movements around things kids love to do, such as running, jumping, climbing, and dancing. This method of approaching the subject of exercise will win the imagination of kids and help them to get fit. The key to remember in designing a workout for children is to keep it fun, fast paced, and maintain a variety of activity. The attention span of children is limited. Allow children to be children. Let the child explore and create an adventure land of movement. Children are naturally drawn to physical activity. The more they do, the more they want to do. Promoting a positive attitude towards fitness instead of *whipping a child into shape,* will create healthy fitness habits that will last a lifetime.

When the "FIT-KIDS" workout program is done at home, the mental and physical characteristics of the child involved must be taken into consideration. Fast, upbeat music can be very helpful in motivating the child to participate in the various fitness activities included in the program. It is essential not to spend more than four minutes on any one particular activity.

Supply the child with some simple props, and plenty of room to move. You will see how creative exercising at an early age can be. Kids don't need expensive equipment to exercise. What they need is an imagination and a few household objects which can turn any house into a fitness center for kids. The following props can easily be obtained to enhance the fitness routine:

- rope
- empty spring water / bottle (thoroughly cleaned)
- dowel sticks (three feet long by three-quarter inch wide)
- wooden stud (two by four)
- aerobic step (if available)
- pom-poms / scarves

- flashlight
- towel
- balloons
- hula hoop
- stop watch
- deck of cards
- chair

- used inner tube (bicycle tire)bleach
- beach ball / volleyball
- cans of soup
- telephone book
- jump-rope
- pillow case

The fitness routine is comprised of four stages. The warm-up stage, the aerobic stage, strengthening activities, and the cool-down. During the warm-up stage, a child should spend approximately ten minutes performing light stretching exercises. This prepares the muscles for more strenuous moves, and guards against injuries. The aerobic stage is considered the endurance segment of activity (I like to call aerobics the "huff and puff" stage). This stage should last approximately twenty to thirty minutes. The idea is to keep moving and have fun. During the strengthening activities, all of the major muscle groups in the arms and legs are exercised to increase the overall strength of the child.

The purpose of the cool-down is to help the body return to a pre-exercise level. Cool-down helps breathing return to normal and keeps muscles from becoming sore and stiff.

The amount of activity completed each day depends upon the fitness level of each individual child. Always encourage, never force children to exercise. Otherwise, they will lose interest in continuing a fitness program.

The following exercises are great for children between the ages of four through eleven. Let these exercises help get them started on a regular fitness routine. You will find versatility within the recommended exercises for your own creativity:

Exercises For Warming-Up and Cooling-Down

- Breathing: Have the children pretend they are balloons. This is done by inhaling deeply, filling the lungs with air, and then exhaling. Repeat several times.

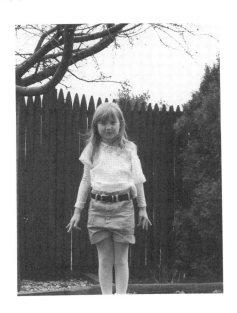 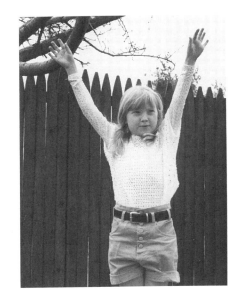

Breathing - Pretending to be a balloon !

• Cheerleading Stretch: Using pom-poms or scarves, wave them up in the air, down towards the floor, to the left, and to the right. Repeat.

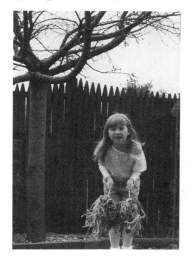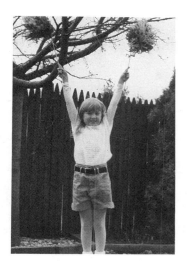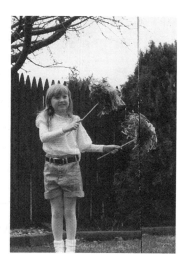

Cheerleading Stretch

• Towel Stretch 1: Stand with feet apart, holding a towel tightly above the head. Slowly stretch to the left, and then to the right. Repeat several times.

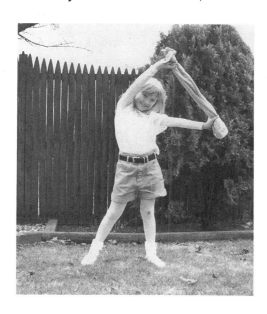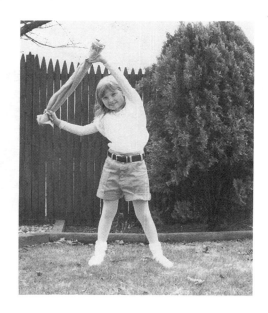

Towel Stretch 1

14

• Towel Stretch 2: Stand with feet apart, holding a towel tightly in front of the body. Slowly twist the upper body to the left, and then to the right.

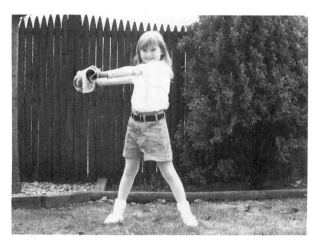

Towel Stretch 2

• Sitting Towel Stretch / Forward Towel Pull: Sit-up with legs stretched-out and straight in front of the body with feet together. Clasp the ends of the towel with each hand. Loop the towel around the soles of the feet. Keep the legs straight and pull the torso forward. Release the stretch. Repeat stretch four times. This warm-up exercise may be performed with one leg at a time. To add variety, bend one leg while keeping the other leg straight.

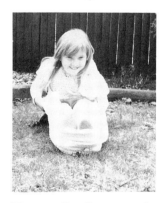 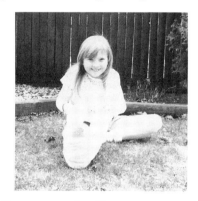

Sitting Towel Stretch / Forward Towel Pull

15

• Stick Twist: Place a stick behind the neck, and clasp the ends of the stick with each hand. While keeping the legs in place, slowly twist the upper body to the left, and then to the right.

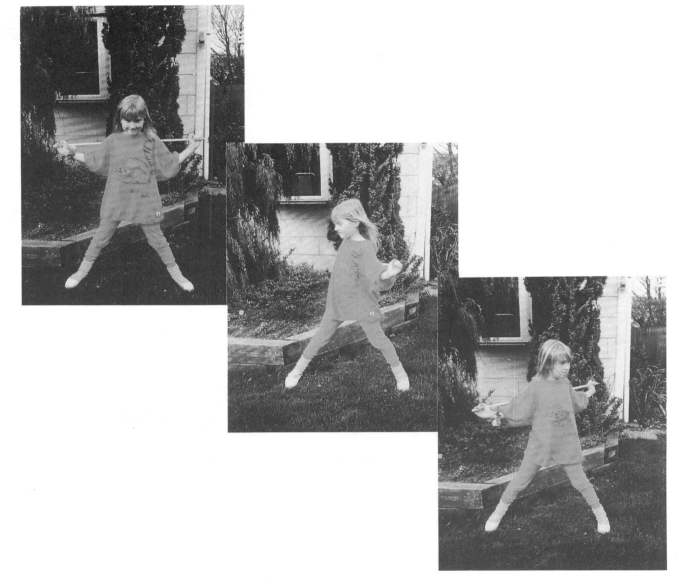

Stick Twist

16

• Stick Kick: Hold a stick at chest level in front of the body, with one hand on each end of the stick. March in place, raising each knee to touch the stick.

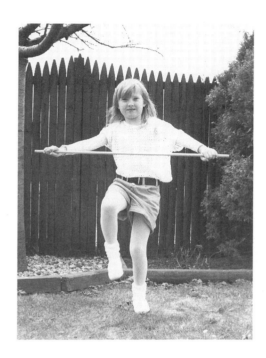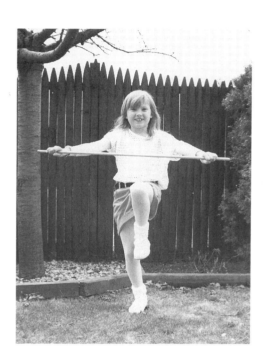

Stick Kick

• Calf Stretch: Place a thick book (i.e., telephone directory) on the floor. Stand with the toes placed on the book, and the heels resting on the floor. Feel the stretch. Raise the heels off the floor, and come up on the toes. Lower the heels back to the floor. Repeat several times.

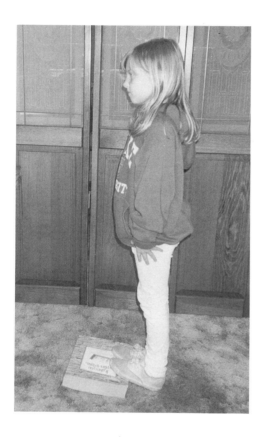 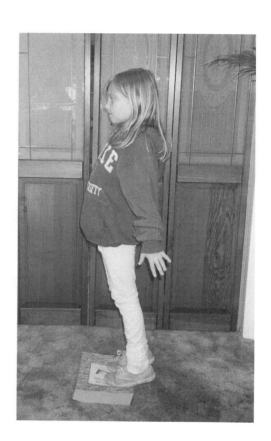

Calf Stretch

Children spend at least six hours a day sitting down in school. Now children can stay in their seats and stretch using the following exercises:

<u>Chair Stretch Work-out</u>

- Sit And Pick: While sitting in a chair, raise each hand and stretch each arm as if picking an apple off a high tree. Alternate each arm, stretching high, then low.

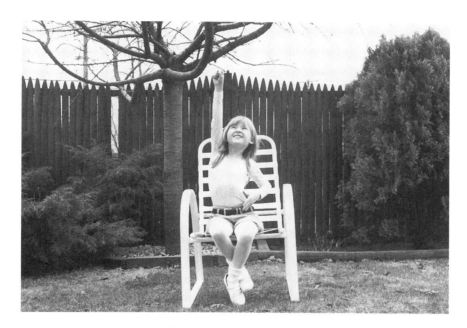

Sit And Pick

• Sit And Swim: Who needs a pool? Just use the arms to simulate a variety of swimming strokes. This may be achieved by rotating the arms forward, and backward. The breast stroke may also be used by pushing the arms together away from the chest, extending all the way forward, separating, and then returning to the sides of the body.

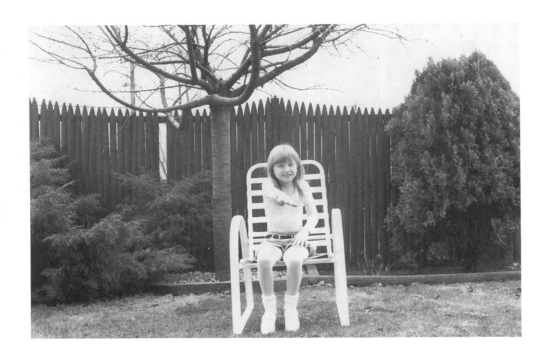

Sit And Swim

• Chair Aerobics: While sitting, bring the right elbow and the left knee together. Then alternate, bringing the left elbow and the right knee together. Repeat several times.

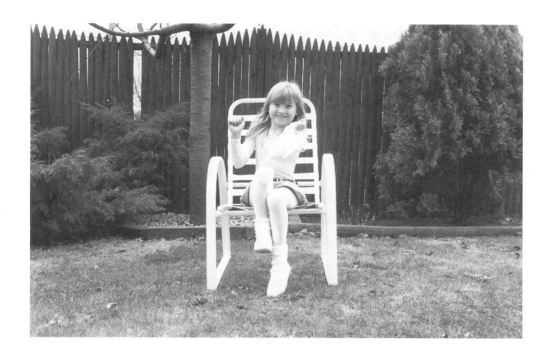

Chair Aerobics

The key to making exercise both fun and effective for children is to create a variety of aerobic activities which will keep them moving. The following exercises have been designed to encourage children to become involved with aerobics:

"Huff And Puff" Aerobic Activities

- T.V. Aerobics: While a child is watching television, the time when a commercial is shown can be beneficial. During each commercial, the child can participate in a "Huff And Puff" aerobic routine of their choice, such as jumping-jacks and jogging in place. With each change of commercial, another activity may be performed.

- "Huff And Puff" Copycat: An exercise game for two or more players which can be played indoors and outdoors. To begin the game, the first child selects and performs an activity. The next child must perform the identical fitness routine in addition to choosing and completing another activity. Each participating child must memorize and complete all of the exercises that were chosen during the game. The "Huff And Puff" Copycat can be fun, aerobic, and is great for improving memory skills.

• Fun-Fit 10 Card Pick-Up: From a deck of playing cards, ten cards are selected at random without exposing their face value. The cards are then placed face-down in strategic areas of the room (select areas which can facilitate a fitness activity). A fitness activity is called out, and a selected child will go to one of the ten cards. The child will turn the card face-up, and perform the number amount of the card (jacks, queens, kings, and aces are counted as ten). For example; if jumping-jacks are called out, and the card turned over is the five of diamonds, the child will perform five jumping-jacks.

• Bring the outdoors in: Your child can have an imaginary playground indoors. This activity can be especially enjoyable when three or children participate. Kids form a circle and begin to jog in place for several seconds. The children jog around the circle several times. Each child stops, lifts an imaginary rope from the ground, and begins to jump rope. After several seconds, the children return to a jog and simulate kicking a soccer ball, or dribbling a basketball. The children can pretend to dribble the ball through their legs and go for a slam dunk. Repeat the entire exercise while remaining in the circle.

Rope has never been so much fun! Listed in this section are several games designed to use pieces of rope in a variety of ways to achieve fitness fun.

- Tic-Tac-Toe String Jump: Place four pieces of rope, four to five feet in length, on the floor. Form the rope into the shape of a tic-tac-toe board. The objective is to have a child stand in the middle square of the board, and jump into as many of the squares as possible with both feet together, during a fifteen second period. A stop-watch can be very helpful in this exercise. The Tic-Tac-Toe String Jump may also use a slight margin of competition.

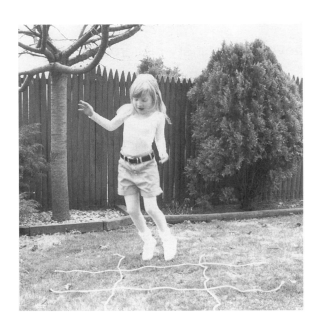 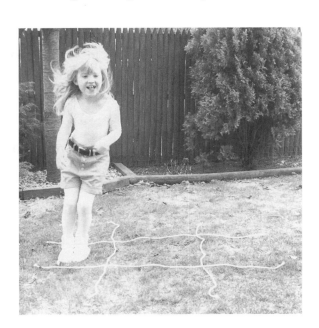

Tic-Tac-Toe String Jump

• Tug-O-War: This game may include two or more players. By using a rope approximately nine feet long, the object is to see which team can pull the opposing team over a designated line. This game is especially useful in strengthening the arms and legs.

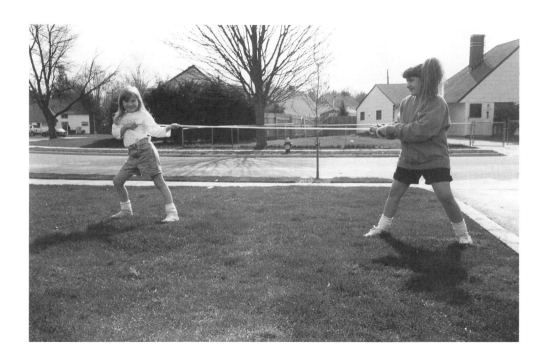

Tug-O-War

• Rope Bridge: By using two chairs and a length of rope approximately nine feet long, a bridge-like structure can be made. Tie the ends of the rope to the backs of the chairs, and adjust the distance between the two chairs. The height of the rope from the floor depends directly on the age and size of the children participating. As the children stand next to the rope, they may take turns in lifting their legs and crossing over to the other side of the rope bridge. This may be repeated several times by crossing over and back again.   Then the child can crawl under, then over. This particular game may be instrumental in toning and strengthening the legs and back.

• Jump To It: Children love to jump rope. Here are some creative ways to help children jump into action; While children are jumping rope, call out various directives, such as; *jump forward, jump backward, jump on one foot / change foot,* and *jog while jumping.*

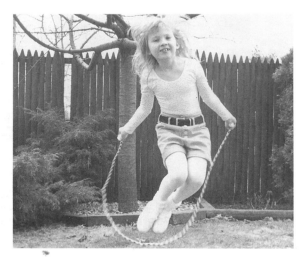

Jump To It

• Fun Jog / Walk: Turn a walk or a jog into an adventure. Ask the child if he or she would like to go for a walk or an adventure, and see which they prefer. A stop-watch can be useful especially if children are allowed to time themselves. It is advisable to begin at a walking pace. A two minute forward walk can be timed, followed with a two minute walk backward. A two minute forward skip may be used as well in addition to a two minute jog. Before you know it, the child has completed a considerable amount of the Fun Walk. The objective is create a fun experience of walking / jogging to the degree that it never resembles a chore. The Fun Walk can be especially enjoyable during the winter season. Children love to make tracks in the snow.

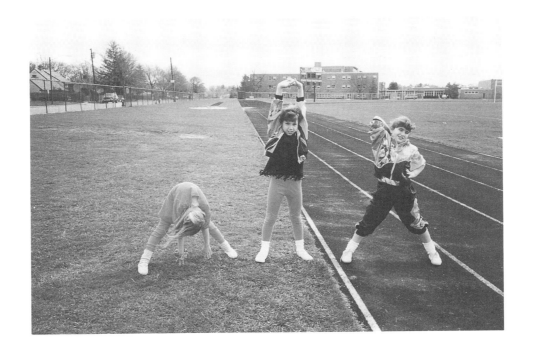

• Olympic Run: It has been found that children love to go to a running track. This experience makes them feel like adults. It is advisable to begin with a walk or a Fun Jog around the track once. Gradually increase the distance each time the track is revisited. A notebook may be very useful to document the progress of children. The information may include the date, the distance, and the amount of time (a stop-watch would then be necessary as well). There may be a section at the bottom of each page (or after every running session) for positive affirmation such as; *"you did great !"* and *"excellent, keep up the good work !"*. This will instill pride of accomplishment and motivation to continue.

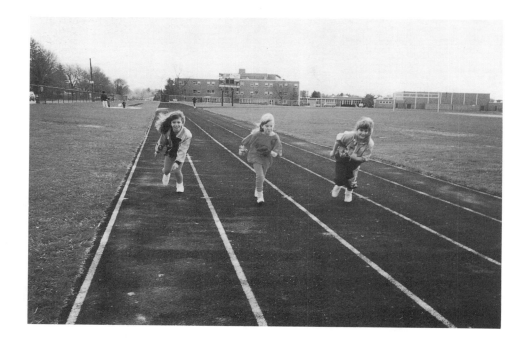

Olympic Run

• Biking: Riding a bicycle has always produced fun times for kids ! This activity should never be discouraged whenever the child has the opportunity. If a stationary bicycle is available (especially during the winter), the child should be encouraged to use it. A stationary bicycle is a great way to workout while watching television.

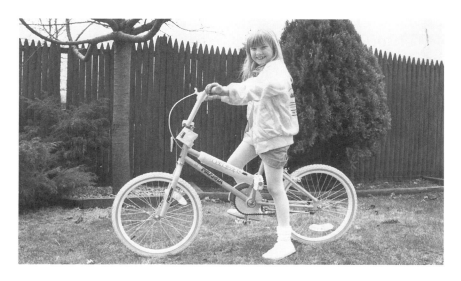

Biking

• Freeze Dance: Best known as a popular park game, the Freeze Dance is also an excellent fitness activity. Basically, the rules are simple. When the music is played, the children begin to dance (more movement means more of an aerobic benefit). When the music stops, the children stop in whatever position they are in, or *freeze* . Another variation of this game can have the children sit-down when the music stops, and stand-up and resume dancing when the music begins again.

• Step To It - Aerobic Step: This particular exercise has become extremely popular with adults. I introduced the aerobic step to the kids that I have worked-out with and it has received overwhelming acceptance. If an aerobic step is available, it can be considered a beneficial addition to the workout program of a child. The step will introduce a fun new dimension to the fitness routine.

When a child begins to use the aerobic step, he or she should be encouraged to march on top of the step. The child can step up and down while waving hands in the air. The child may also turn sideways and perform a side step routine. To add some spice into a step program, have the child bounce a small ball on the step while stepping up and down. There are many variations of exercise while using the aerobic step. The best way to motivate a child to become involved with the aerobic step is to participate in the activity together.

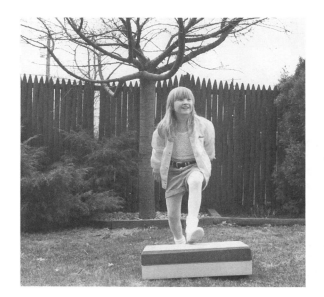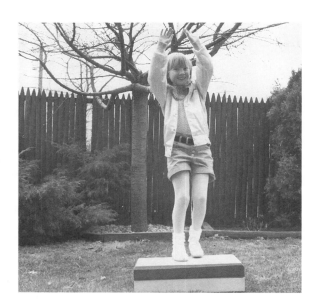

Step To It

STRENGTHENING EXERCISE FUN

Hula Craze

• Hula Hoop: The hula hoop is a great fitness toy. It may used in the conventional way which is to spin the hoop around the waist. Contests can be held on who can spin it the longest. The hula hoop may also be used on the arms and legs.   It is important to be creative when designing a fitness program. The hula hoop enables creativity because of it's versatility.

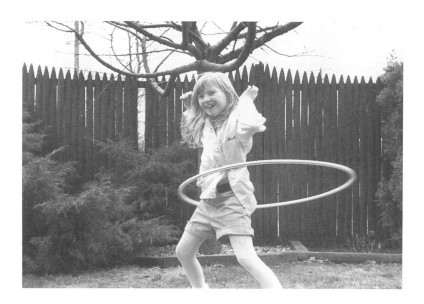

• Hula Tumble: Using adult supervision, a child can perform forward rolls.

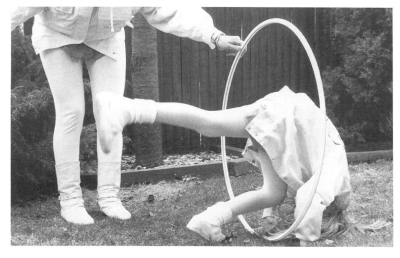

• Hula Throw: The hula hoop may be held from the sides in an upright position, to be used for a bean bag or ball toss.

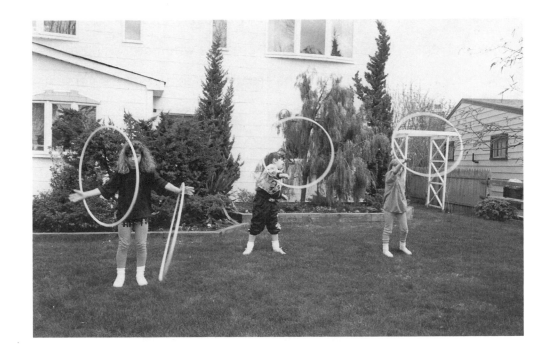

• Hula Hula Holler: A large area is required for this exercise game (outdoors is an ideal place). Two or more children can play. With hula hoops placed strategically on the ground, music is played. The children begin to run / skip around the hoops. When the music is stopped, the children jump into a hoop closest to them and spin it around the waist, leg, or arm. The game is resumed when the music is started again.

• Balance Beam (with hula hoop): A balance beam can be easily simulated by using a two-by-four piece of wood (approximately eight feet in length. be extremely effective in the development of coordination. A hula hoop can be used to create a more challenging exercise. An adult may hold the hula hoop over the balance beam. A child can then walk through the hoop while on the balance beam. A variation of this exercise may include walking on all fours, or even crawling.

With additional supervision, a dowel stick may be included in the exercise. After the child has walked through the hula hoop, he or she may walk over the dowel stick (the distance of the dowel stick over the balance beam should be adjusted in accordance with the age and size of the child). This exercise may be repeated as the child walks to the end of the balance beam and turns around . The child may also try to spin the hula hoop around the waist while walking across the balance beam.

Other props that may be used on the balance beam are jacks and a clothes pin. The jacks may be placed on one end of the balance beam. The child will then assume a duck walk position. The object of the exercise is to attempt to pick up as many jacks as possible with the clothes pin, duck walk to the other side of the balance beam, and safely deliver the jacks. This can be used in a competitive manner as well. However, safety should be recognized at all times. This particular exercise strengthens the legs and increases coordination.

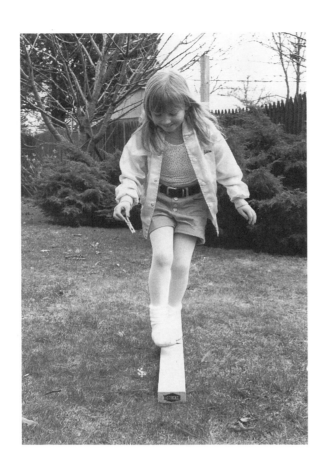

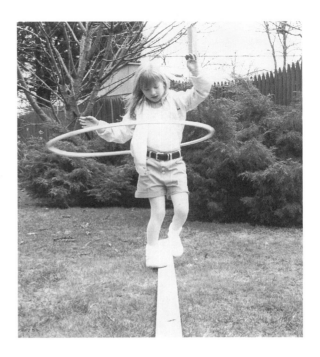

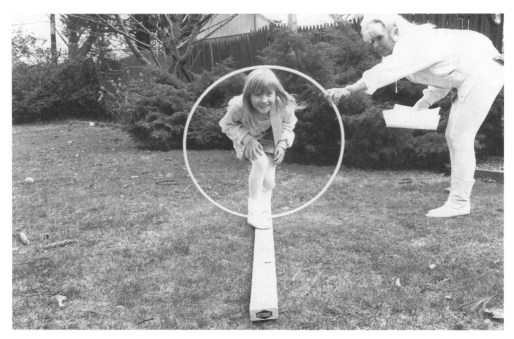

Balance Beam With Hula Hoop

34

- Flashlight Dance: One or two flashlights may be used in a spacious room (it is not necessary to decrease the ambient lighting of the room). Shine the light(s) onto the floor, and encourage the child to jump onto the spot light. Keep changing the position of the light, and have the child jump onto each new position. The light may also be shined onto the walls. The child can reach for the light with their arms. This activity will strengthen arms and legs, and increase coordination.

- Weight-Lifting With Bottles: Emptied one gallon bottles (spring water or bleach bottles for example) may be filled with water or sand. The amount that is filled can be altered to create different weights. The children can hold the bottles at their sides, and slowly curl their arms towards their chests. With the bottles held at the sides. The child can bend the elbows and raise the bottles simulating a bird in flight. To strengthen the triceps, have the child use only one bottle at a time. He or she can lean forward and extend an arm backward. These exercise will strengthen arms and shoulders.

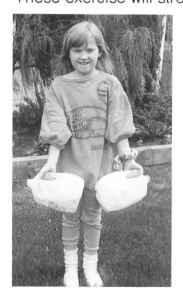 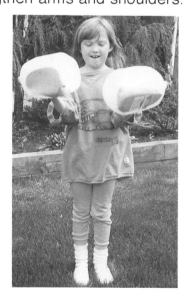 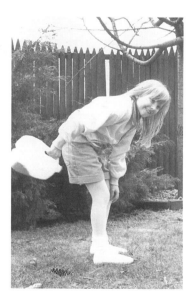

Weight-Lifting With Bottles

35

• Pole Rock: In this particular activity, a child is given a dowel stick while music is played. There is a variety of exercises that may be performed. For example, while holding the dowel stick in front of them in a horizontal position, the child can begin with knee lifts (lightly touching the stick). The child may also raise the dowel stick above their head, and slowly twist their upper body to the left, and then to the right. The dowel stick may also be used to simulate an air guitar to the music. *"Rocking the night away"* can be used as a valuable aerobic benefit.

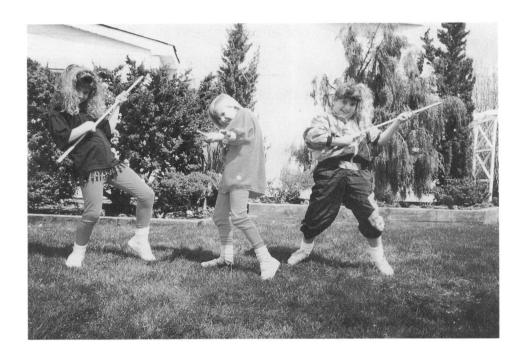

Pole Rock

What do you usually do with the inner tube of a bicycle when it becomes old or punctured beyond repair? Throw it out? Not anymore. The inner tube can be used as a great piece of exercise equipment. The size of the child should be taken into consideration when selecting the proper sized inner tube. However, the size of any inner tube can be modified to become proportionate to the child. This may be done simply by cutting one section of the tube, then tie the ends closer together. The following exercises utilize the bicycle inner tube:

- Sit-Down Row: Sit-up with legs stretched-out and straight in front of the body with feet together. Hold onto the inner tube with each hand. Loop the inner tube around the soles of the feet. While keeping the legs straight, pull the inner tube toward the chest. Release the stretch. Repeat this motion, and row, row, row.

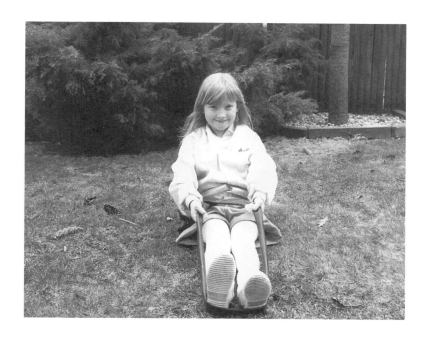

Sit-Down Row

37

- Biceps Pull: Children can build strength in the arms, chest, and shoulders with this activity. Place a section of the inner tube under the soles of the feet and stand straight up. With palms open and facing up, clasp one side of the inner tube with each hand. Slowly, curl one arm at a time toward the chest. Slowly, return the arms to the original position (straight down in front of the body). This exercise may be repeated several times and may be increased with time as endurance increases.

- Waist Workout: The child can trim and strengthen their waist by placing a section of the inner tube underneath the soles of the feet while standing. With palms open and facing up, clasp one side of the inner tube with each hand. Slowly, bend to the left, then to the right.

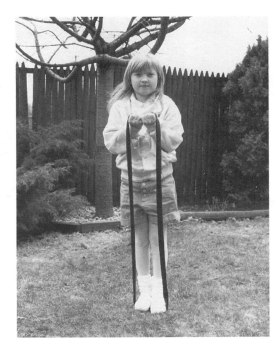

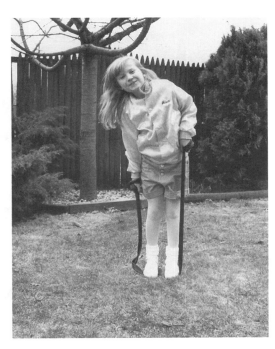

Biceps Pull   Waist Workout

The following strength building activities can easily be performed by turning cans of soup or books into homemade dumbbells:

• Biceps Curl: This particular activity can be done in a standing position or while seated in a straight- backed chair. Hold a can of soup or a book of equal weight in each hand. Slowly, curl the arms towards the chest. Slowly, return the arms straight down to the front of the body. This exercise may also be repeated several times and may be increased with time as endurance increases.

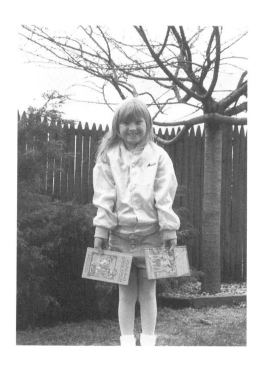 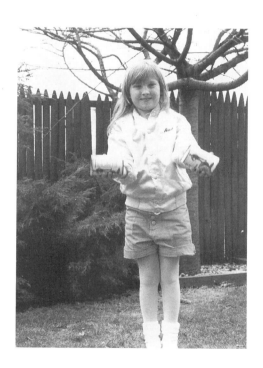

Biceps Curl

• Triceps: The muscles in the back of the upper arm, the triceps, may also be strengthened by using cans of soup or books. Hold a can of soup or a book in one hand (only one arm at a time will be exercised). Lean forward while in a sitting position, or bend forward while standing (it may be necessary to support the upper body by leaning onto a table when standing). Extend the arm backward slowly. Then return the arm forward to the original position. This exercise may also be repeated several times and may be increased with time as endurance increases.

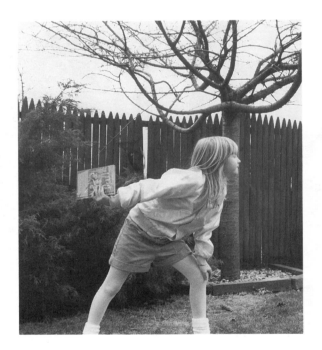 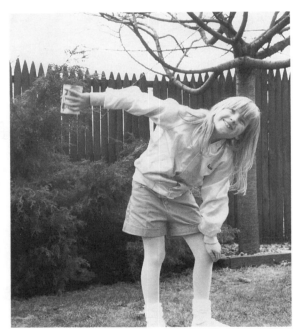

Triceps

40

Balloons are not just for parties anymore when they can be turned into exercise equipment! Balloons are an excellent way to teach kids how to strengthen muscles. The following exercises illustrate how balloons can assist in the FIT-KID Workout.

Use a standard nine-inch balloon. An adult should inflate and tie the balloon at approximately three-quarter capacity. The child should be able to feel the resistance of the air pressure without bursting the balloon.

• Chest and Arms: Place hands flat on both sides of the balloon in front of the body while standing. Squeeze and release several times.

Another variation of this exercise would be to hold the balloon between the elbows while standing. Squeeze and release several times.

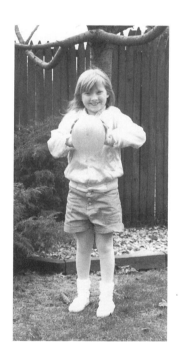 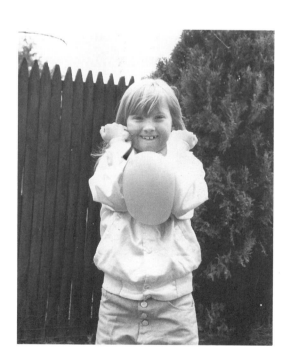

Balloon Squeeze For Chest & Arms

• Lat Squeeze (upper back): Have the child hold one balloon on each side of the body between the elbow and waist. Press elbow into balloon and waist. Hold and release. Repeat several times.Imitating animals can be a favorite pastime of children.

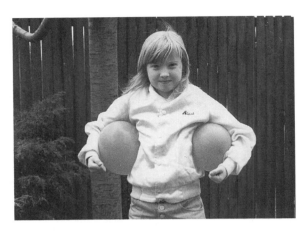

Lat Squeeze

• Inner Thigh Strengthener: Have the child sit on the floor with knees bent and feet flat on the floor. Place balloon between the knees while leaning back with palms also flat on the floor. Squeeze the knees together several times.

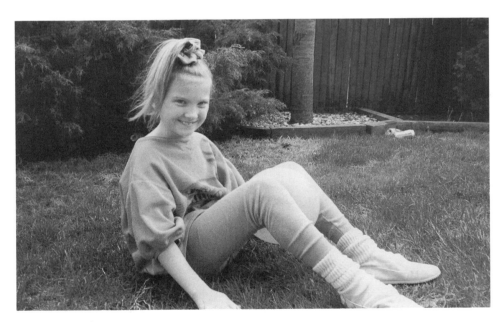

Inner Thigh Strengthener

42

• Rear Upper Leg (hamstring): Have the child stand up straight and hold the back of a chair. Place the balloon behind one knee and bring the heel toward the backside. Squeeze and release. Do not release completely, otherwise the balloon will become loose. Repeat several times.

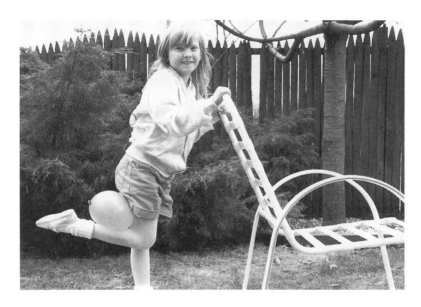

Rear Upper Leg (hamstring)

• Body Rock Balloon Bop: One or more children can play. A balloon is tossed into the air (children may stand in a circle). The object of the game is to keep the balloon up in the air by hitting it with body parts (elbows, head, knees, etc.). Don't let it hit the floor. Keep moving!

The following section describes how it easy it can become to motivate children by using *ANIMAL ACTION, Turning Children Into Fit Animals* :

- Leap Frog: Squat down to the floor. While placing most of the weight on the heels, rest hands in front of the body on the floor. Leap forward as high as possible. This activity strengthens the legs.

- Bunny Rabbit: Hop, hop, hop! The child could imitate a little bunny by hopping around on both legs, and then one leg at a time. This activity also strengthens the legs.

- Cat Crawl: During this exercise, the child walks on all fours. This activity will strengthens the arms, legs, shoulders, and back.

- Crab Crawl: This activity is similar to the Cat Crawl, however, the child leans backward on all fours (the front of the body faces toward the ceiling). Walking around like a crab will strengthen other muscles of the arms, legs, shoulders, and back.

- Jumping Kangaroo: Have the child pretend they are a kangaroo. Jumping in place is a good beginning. Various commands can be shouted out, such as "jump side-to-side", "jump forward", and "jump backward" for example.

• Bird In Flight: Have the child lean forward slightly and place a small pillow on the back of the neck. With hands stretched-out from the sides, the child can pretend to fly around the room while balancing the pillow. This activity promotes a sense of balance and coordination.

• Worm: During this particular activity, the child imitates a worm wiggling across the floor. In order to achieve this, the child will lay down on the (with the back in contact with the floor). By using only the buttocks, back, and shoulders, the child will wiggle across the floor. Avoiding the use of the hands on the floor will create a more beneficial exercise.

• Lame Sparrow: In this exercise, the child can pretend to be a poor little sparrow which has a broken leg. The sparrow now has only one leg to get around with. The child can hop around on one leg while holding the other leg up with one hand. The hopping leg should be alternated when necessary. The strengthening benefits for the legs are obvious in this activity. But the coordination which is developed is also very important.

The following section describes how to motivate children by having them imagine they are participating in sports activities. The activities which are mentioned are excellent ways to inspire a child to pursue the actual sport as well.

Sports Imagination Style

- Shadow Boxing: The children can imagine they are prize fighters. Without making physical contact with anything (including other children), the moves of a fighter can be imitated. Jabs, hooks, crosses, bobbing, and weaving are all part of the fun! An excellent aerobic activity, as well as a strength and confidence builder. Playing the theme from ROCKY will motivate the kids to become more involved in this activity also.

- Tennis: Children can imagine they are participating in a tennis game. He or she may practice an overhand serve, a return shot, or their backhand. Placement of feet may also be practiced as well as starting, stopping, and pivoting.

- Baseball: An entire baseball game can be simulated. The children can pretend to hit a home run, and run to three bases located around the room, Eventually making it back to home plate!

- Basketball: Children may pretend to play the game of basketball. By using any lightweight inflatable ball which is proportionate to the size of the child or just pretending to have a ball, it is easy to play an imaginary game of basketball. The children can practice dribbling the ball to an imaginary basket. Have the children alternate dribbling the ball with their left and right hands. Dribbling the ball behind the back and between the legs is an excellent way to develop coordination.

- Popcorn Popping Play: Have children imagine they are corn kernels, starting in a crouched position on the floor. Then have them jump up high, as if they were popping like popcorn.

- Giant / Small Walk: Instruct the children to stand tall and begin walking. After they have taken several steps, instruct them to slowly bend the knees and continue to walk into a squat position. Then have the children slowly walk back up to a standing position. Repeat several times. This exercise will help to strengthen the legs.

- Ball Squeeze: In a sitting position, the child may place a beach ball or a volley ball between the legs. Instruct the child to squeeze the ball, then release the tension. This activity will increase strength of the inner thighs.

- Ball Jump: This particular exercise is a variation of the Ball Squeeze. Instead, the child begins the activity in a standing position. As the ball is squeezed between the legs, the child will begin to hop around the room without dropping the ball. This activity increases leg strength and coordination.

47

• Pillow Case Race: This activity is a variation of the potato sack race. A large pillow case will be needed for this activity. Have the child stand inside the pillow case clasping the sides of the case with both hands. The child may begin hopping from one side of the room to the other. Adult supervision is advised for this activity. This exercise will help develop the balance and coordination as well the leg muscles of the child.

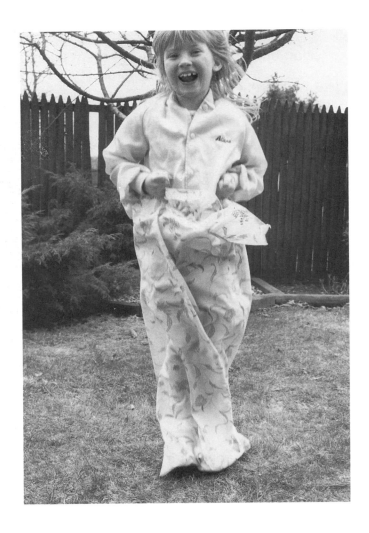

Pillow Case Race

48

• Mattress Workout: Children naturally see every bed as a trampoline. Therefore, why not allow them to practice jumping to their hearts content. Place the mattress onto a cleared area of the floor. With adult supervision, children may begin to perform *amazing* moves! This exercise will increase leg strength.

• Roam the *Make Believe* Balance Beam: With several two-by-four pieces of wood, it is easy to simulate a balance beam in a zig-zag formation. Place the beams of wood onto a cleared area of the floor. The child can pretend to be a gymnast by walking across the beams forward, sideways, and backward. The child may even try to balance a book on top of the head while walking. This activity shall help develop balance and coordination, and create a lot of fun!

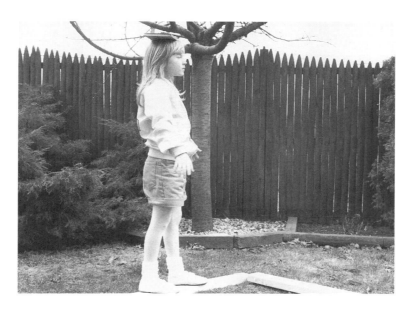

Roam the Make Believe Balance Beam

• Ski Slalom: An addition to the make believe balance beam can be the use of a balloon to simulate a ski slalom. Have the child place the balloon between the legs and squeeze while jumping from one side of the balance beam to the other. Once the child has reached the end, they can turn around travel back to the starting point the same way.

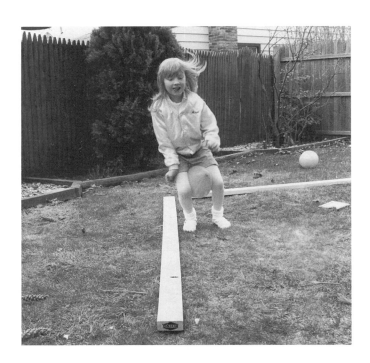

Ski Slalom

• Hop Scotch: If there isn't an area already designated for the game of Hop Scotch, the child may still pretend to play. The child can jump forward with two feet, then hop with one foot. The child may alternate between one and two legged jumps. This exercise will help develop balance and coordination as well the leg muscles.

• Wall Sit: Have the child stand with the back firmly against the wall. The child may begin to slowly bend the knees while sliding the back down the wall until a pretend sitting position is achieved. The child is then seated in a imaginary chair. Hold this position for fifteen seconds. This exercise may be repeated several times to develop strength in the thigh muscles.

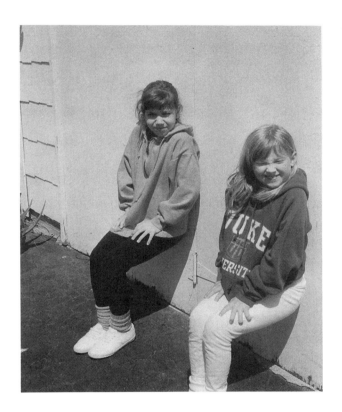

Wall Sit

• Wall Push-Ups: Similar to conventional push-ups performed on the floor, the wall push-up may be slightly easier for a child to perform. The child may stand one arm's length in front of a wall. By placing the hands approximately two feet apart, the child may lean on the wall while keeping the arms straight. Slowly, the child may bend the arms and lean closer toward the wall. Have the child attempt to touch the nose to the wall, and then return to the original position (by straightening the elbow). This exercise may be repeated several times to strengthen arms and chest muscles.

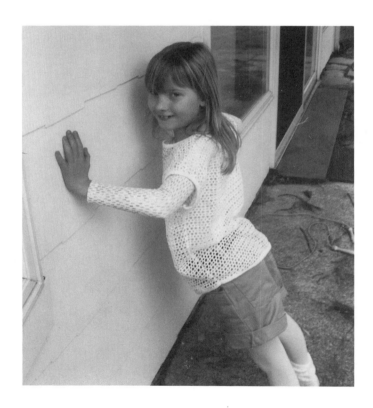

Wall Push-Ups

52

• Upside-down Bike Race: The child can lay on the back and place the legs in the air. The bed or a padded area of the floor may be suitable areas chosen for this activity. The child can pretend to pedal an imaginary bicycle. The speed may alternate between slow, moderate, and fast.

• AB Crunch: The child can lay on the back with hands placed behind the head and the knees bent (feet flat on the floor). Have the child curl into a ball, then return to the original position. This exercise may be repeated several times as it will strengthen the abdominal muscles.

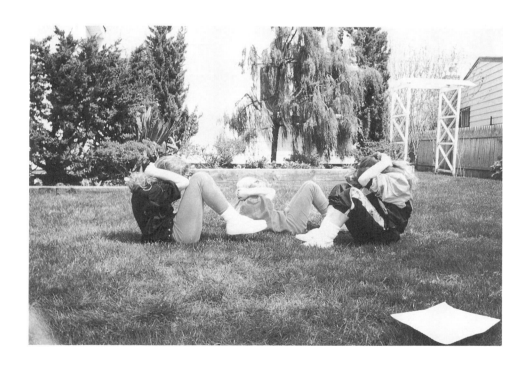

AB Crunch

• Peek-A-Boo: The child can lay on the back and place the legs in the air in a "V" position. A padded area of the floor is advisable for this activity. The child may lift the shoulders forward and bring the hands through the legs. The child may then return to the original position. This exercise may be repeated several times as it will also strengthen the abdominal muscles.

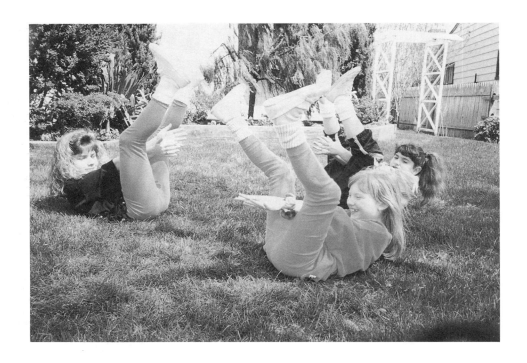

Peek-A-Boo

• Siamese Twins: Have two children sit back-to-back on the floor with their arms locked together. Both children should keep their knees bent and feet flat on the floor. Simultaneously, both children should press firmly against each other and begin to stand up. This activity may be performed several times in order to strengthen the legs.

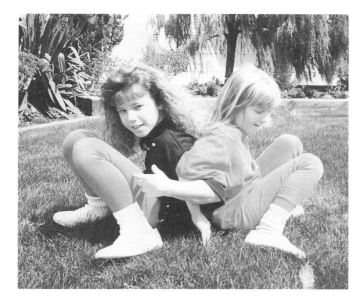
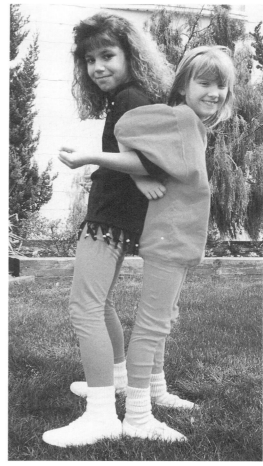

Siamese Twins

- Drawbridge: Have two children lie flat on their backs in a toe-to-toe formation. Have the children lift their legs into the air and place the soles of their feet together. Slowly, the children can straighten their legs and use resistance to lift their backs off the floor and rest on their shoulders. The position may be held for several seconds. Then the children may slowly decrease the resistance and lower their backs. This activity may be performed several times.

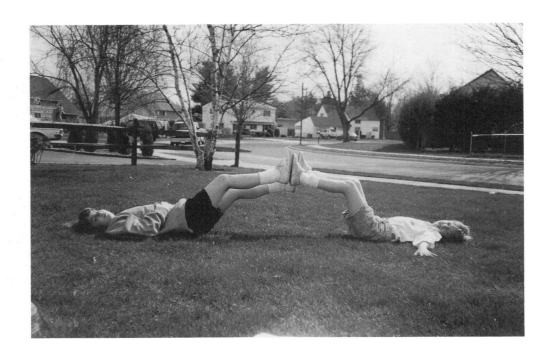

Drawbridge

• Bicycle for 2: This activity is similar to the drawbridge. Have two children lie flat on their backs in a toe-to-toe formation. Have the children lift their legs into the air and place the soles of their feet together.   The children may then use an alternating resistance against their partner's feet. Pedaling together, the children should push from the thighs while holding the stomach tight.

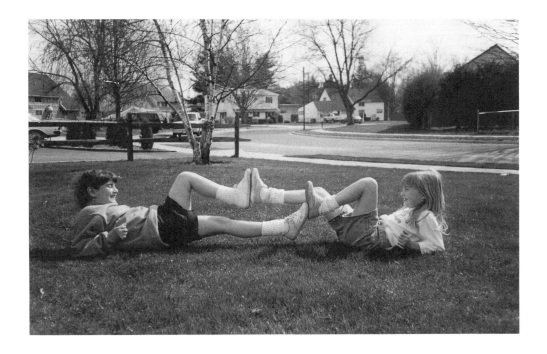

Bicycle for 2

• Skiers: In this activity, have the children stand and face each other while holding hands with their arms straight. Slowly, both children may begin to lower themselves toward the floor until they reach a squatting position (a skier's tucked position). Then, slowly, both children may begin to pull themselves back up to a standing position.

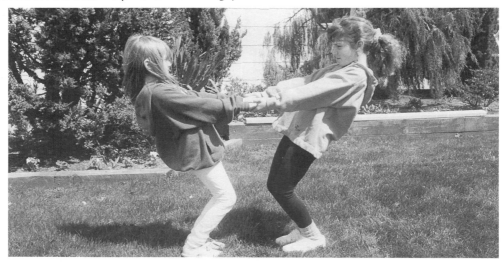

Skiers

• Row-Row-Row The Boat: Have two children sit on the floor while facing each with their legs spread apart and their toes touching. With their arms straight in front of them, have the children hold hands. The children may begin to alternate leaning forward, then backward simulating a rowing boat.

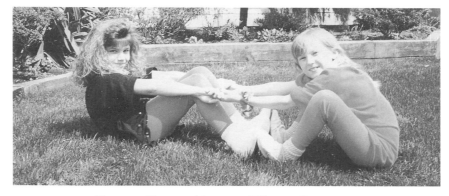

Row-Row-Row The Boat

58

EXERCISE IDEAS FOR FAMILY FITNESS (or a group of kids)

Relay Races: Children will continue to enjoy this activity as long as creative and challenging relays are introduced. In order to establish organization, teams will have to be formed. The first person on each team will race toward a turn around point (wall, tree, chair, etc.) then race back to the line and tag the next person on the team. The first team to have all of their players return to the starting line wins. It is very important to make sure that all the teams are evenly matched. The following are just a few ways to develop relay races:

- Walk as fast as possible balancing an egg on a spoon without dropping it.
- Balance a book on the top of the head while racing toward the goal, and return running on all fours.
- Dribble a ball with hands toward the goal and back.
- Run backwards both ways.
- Skip.
- Jump rope toward the goal and back.
- Hop on both feet toward the goal, and return hopping on one foot.

Obstacle Courses: The entire family can become involved in developing a challenging obstacle course. An obstacle course can be created from a backyard gym or at a park. Take advantage of natural obstacles such as trees, stumps, etc.). The obstacle course is an excellent way to improve cardiovascular conditioning and strength.

The following samples illustrate just a few ways an obstacle course can be created:

- Skip to the landmark, touch it, then hop through a series of hula hoops or tires.
- Zig-zag through a maze of cones or other objects.
- Crawl through a tunnel made with a sheet and chairs.
- Walk across a two-by-four balance beam (placed on the ground) forward and backward.
- Jump over strings placed across the floor.
- Sprint to the finish line.

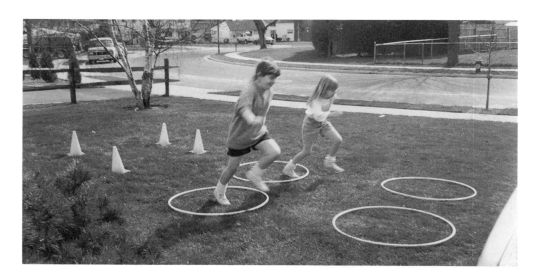

Obstacle Course

• Circuit Circus: This activity is a method of circuit training for children. In order to set up the circuit circus, many of the exercises previously mentioned may be selected. You may even choose to design your own activities and incorporate them into the circuit. The child should spend at least two minutes at each workout station, and then proceed to the next activity.

SAMPLE OF A 12 MINUTE CIRCUIT

(The amount of time and quantity of activities may be varied)

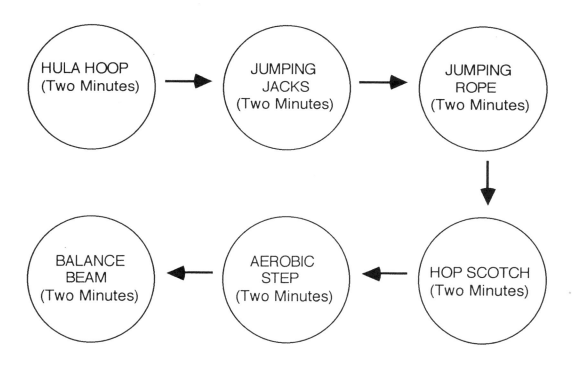

Exercise should become a habit. There are several ways to achieve this. The more routine you can make it, the better chance that it will become an daily occurrence. Create a special place indoors and outdoors where exercise can be performed. Also, try to exercise the same time every day. Incorporate as much consistency around exercise as possible so that it becomes part of the day, and not something rare. There is no better time than when children are young to get them hooked on fitness fun!

- Always remember to encourage the child to drink plenty of fluids when working-out.
- Never push the child to workout. When the child becomes tired, allow him or her to stop and rest.

FIT-KIDS: GETTING KIDS "HOOKED" ON FITNESS FUN!

CHAPTER 5
FAMILY FITNESS

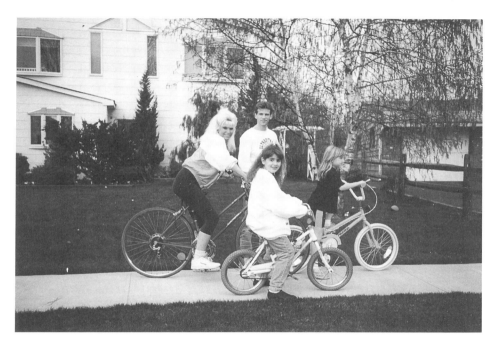

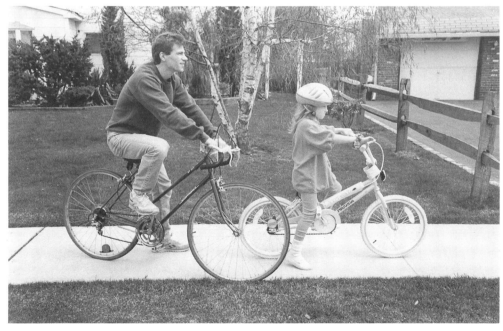

Five

A family that exercises together, becomes fit together. The best way for a family to get started is to launch a Family Fitness Program. Constant participation and interest in such a program will reinforce the entire family's commitment to become fit.

Family fitness can begin when one or both parents share in related activities. The activities selected should be designed to instill enjoyment to everyone involved. This chapter may be used as a guideline when creating Family Fitness Program.

Steps For A Family Fitness Program

Step One: The family can be gathered together to discuss the type of activities everyone can participate in. When exploring options, it is a good idea to select activities which could assist the family in becoming aerobically fit. An activity that causes you to move steadily for at least twenty to thirty minutes would be considered aerobic. Examples of aerobic activities are walking, jogging, playing tennis, swimming, skiing, and bicycling.

Step Two: Establish a routine. Develop an activity plan which incorporates at least three days a week. It is important to rotate the types of activities to ensure variety and avoid boredom. Parents may find it particularly difficult to maintain this type of program with busy work schedules. It may be necessary to have each parent select one day of the week (late afternoon, early evening). During the weekend, the entire family can join together for an activity. With an arrangement such as the one mentioned, everyone can enjoy the fitness benefits. Moreover, parents will be spending quality time with their children.

Step Three: Introduce a Wall Chart Of Success. A progress chart which illustrates the fitness accomplishments of each family member. This particular tool can be invaluable in stimulating a greater appreciation of the Family Fitness Program. A more detailed explanation of the Wall Chart Of Success is supplied in chapter seven with a sample chart.

Step Four: Implement an award system. Distributing awards will provide added incentives for children. A ribbon of achievement, certificate, or small trophy may be purchased at a stationary or party supply store. These types of awards can be given on a weekly or monthly basis. Chapter nine, Rewarding The Fitness Process, describes in more detail how the award system can play an integral part of instilling motivation.

Step Five: Proper nutrition for the family must accompany any fitness program. Establish correct eating habits for children from the beginning. Part three of this book will detail various aspects of nutrition, which will help the entire family on the road to healthy eating.

When pursuing family fitness activities, it is important to remember to take one day at a time. While exercising and eating right, everyone is achieving an improved physical condition gradually. The entire process should should remain enjoyable in order to obtain the best results.

The following activities are designed to produce results, and keep everyone involved interested while continuing to have fun!

Adventure Walk

Walking is an excellent family fitness idea. It requires no special equipment with the exception of sneakers, and it can be done almost anywhere. Walking is a great cardiovascular exercise which improves the condition of the heart and helps to decrease body fat. Most of the major muscle groups are utilized when walking. It also assists in reducing stress and increasing one's energy level.

At times, it may be difficult to get a child to go out for a walk. Since there are so many forms of transportation available today, walking may appear to be a chore. But if you suggest to take an *Adventure Walk* with the child (or children), the entire way a child perceives walking, could change for life.

When taking an *Adventure Walk,* you and the child can search for pine cones, fallen leaves of particular colors, or tracks in the dirt or snow. During part of the walk, you and the child can take turns hopping, skipping, and walking backward. Everyone can help turn an average walk into a fun filled event.

A consideration may be the purchase of a stopwatch. The style of walking can be monitored. At every one or two minute interval, the type of walk can be changed. If the child was to wear the stopwatch around his or her neck, they would realize a new found sense of responsibility and maturity. In the same frame of thought, a whistle may also be used as a valuable prop (as long as the privilege isn't misused). Walking, as an activity, may be included in a family journal or on the Wall Chart Of Success (detailed in chapter seven).

Family Biking

Purchasing bicycles for the entire family is a wise investment for health. Bicycling with children should begin when the child is approximately eight to nine months old. The baby can ride in custom infant seat secured to the back of the parents bicycle. The child will grow to love bicycling when exposed to an exercise environment at an early age.

When planning a family biking trip, make sure that all family members wear helmets. Also, the pace of bicycling should be maintained to accommodate the slowest family member.

The child should be allowed to assist in the planning of a bike outing. When initially starting, choose an easy trip (mostly level and only two to five miles). After several trips, the course may be extended in gradual increments.

Health Club Visit

As a Director of a health club on Long Island, New York, I was able to offer *FAMILY FITNESS DAYS* to members. A special program in which all family members are welcome to participate on the various exercises. This included aerobic classes, the use of stationary bicycles, treadmills, rowing machines, stair climbing equipment, and universal weight training.

With proper supervision and guidance, children and parents alike have benefited greatly from this program. If you are presently a member of a health club, it would be advantages to discuss this idea with the health club manager or director.

T. V. Time Converted Into Productive Time

If there is a VCR available, renting several exercise tapes is a unique way of altering the focus of the child whom is fixated on watching television. Interacting with the exercise videos allows the child to satisfy the habit of watching television in addition to becoming healthy. Parents and educators alike can utilize this form of exercise participation, especially with the wide variety of videos presently available. Moreover, this can be a great time for mother and child to have a special workout together.

There are many aspects to a *FAMILY FITNESS PROGRAM* aside from the physical benefits. Family members that exercise together have much more to share and enjoy better communication. This results in an overall better relationship.

Exercising together can alleviate tension in children and adults alike. It can also be the perfect time to discuss the various aspects of the life of the child.

When becoming involved in a *FAMILY FITNESS PROGRAM*, an adult should learn to play as a child. Be silly, and have some fun. Fitness require discipline, but not stress. It is extremely important to instill fun into every activity. Otherwise, the child will be influenced to believe that exercise causes anger or other negative emotions.

Family fitness makes a lot of sense when there is a need for a healthy change. Support by family members is a key factor when promoting changes in habit. Beginning a *FAMILY FITNESS PROGRAM* is an excellent method of having the entire family spend quality time together while staying healthy.

Give the children a gift that will last a lifetime; the gift of staying fit and healthy.

FIT-KIDS: GETTING KIDS "HOOKED" ON FITNESS FUN!

CHAPTER 6

IT'S A PARTY!

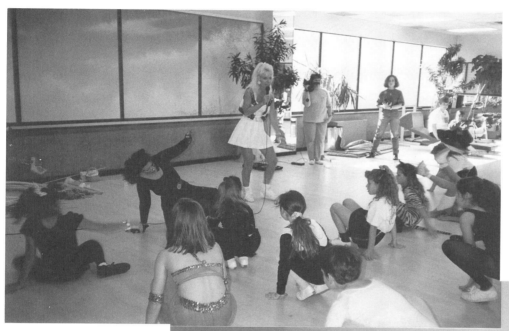

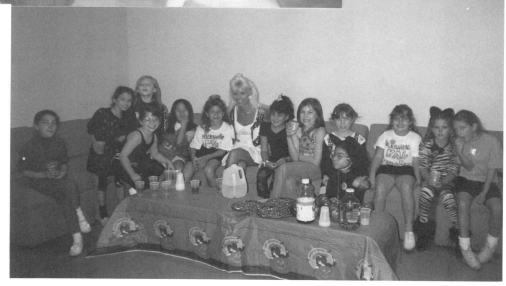

Six

When planning a *FIT-KID PARTY* , deciding the date, time , place, and the length of the party is extremely important. The date should be when most of the invited children will be available (usually during the weekend). The time when the party is given depends on meals will be served (snacks, lunch, or dinner).

Make sure that wherever a *FIT-KID PARTY* is held, there must be plenty of room available to move around. Some examples of *FIT-KID PARTY* locations are large basements (uncluttered), backyards, or even a rented party room.

A common question is "How long should a *FIT-KID PARTY* last?". Most parties for children do not exceed one-and-a-half to two hours. This is usually ample time for children to achieve a healthy work-out while still having fun, and not get getting "burned-out".

A guest list and creative invitations should be the next part of the *FIT-KID PARTY* plan. Invitations set the mood and sometimes the theme for the party. They help to create enthusiasm for the party. Whether you choose to purchase invitations, or make them yourself, the element of energy and motivation should be present.

If you are creating your own invitation, you may choose to cut colored construction paper into the shape of a sneaker. Another idea you may pursue is the placement of fitness stickers onto post cards (be sure to leave enough room on the cards for vital party information).

When writing the invitation itself, make sure that the wording is absolutely clear. It is very common to forget a vital piece of information such as a date, address, or directions.

An especially fun idea prior to sealing the invitation into an envelope is the addition of confetti or glitter. This has a magical affect when the envelope is opened, and the invitation is removed, the confetti will fly out. This type of invitation will surely be remembered.

A consideration which should be used is the amount of advance notice required. Make sure you send out the invitations at least three weeks before hand. This practice will avoid any conflict of schedules from occurring with any other parties.

Now that you have completed the selection of the date, time, location, length of party, guest list, and invitation format. It is now time to create a list of party goods needed. I have supplied several guidelines which can be used to customize your very own *FIT-KID PARTY* .

1) **Decorations** always add life to a party. Balloons and streamers are extremely effective. A few extra balloons on hand are invaluable when conducting fitness games.

2) Cups, plates, and utensils: Using paper and plastic goods ensure safety and make cleaning-up much easier. Bright colored cups, plates, and utensils are more appealing to the eyes. As an addition, attractive toothpicks and umbrella sticks for finger foods may be used. Multi-colored straws can add a new dimension of interest when serving juice. More guidelines can be read in chapter fourteen, Food Fit For A Kid.

3) Food: Selecting the type of food to serve depends on what time of day the *FIT-KID PARTY* is being held. Remember, it is very important to keep the emphasis on providing healthy foods. A *FIT-KID BUFFET* may be considered to be the perfect alternative the same old pizza and hot dogs. Many buffet ideas are also highlighted in chapter fourteen.

4) Dessert: Try to be imaginative when serving dessert. A frozen yogurt bar / buffet may be a better choice instead of ice cream and cake. This can be achieved with several bowls filled with favorite toppings such as raisins, granola, banana slices, strawberry slices, lite chocolate syrup, and lite whipped cream. Supply each child with a large colorful, disposable cup filled with frozen yogurt. The children can select which toppings they prefer.

5) "Goodie-bags" and Prizes: Most parties have "goodie-bags" as going home presents as well as prizes for games. Everyone should go home a winner. Candy should not be used as a prize unless it's sugar-free. Here are some creative ideas for *FIT-KID PARTY* "goodie-bags";

• jump rope • jacks • balls • stickers • hula hoops.

If you want to make a goody give-away that is quite original, small white or colored irregular towels can be purchased inexpensively. The towels can be used to wrap a fitness toy. This can be accomplished by rolling the fitness prize in the towel, and tying it with a large ribbon. The children can be told that the towel is to be used for future work-outs.

As an added bonus, tell the children in the beginning of the *FIT-KID PARTY*, that exercising awards will be distributed. Children love to take home a ribbon of achievement or a plastic trophy.

Planning the actual *FIT-KID PARTY WORKOUT* will require some preparation. Arrange to have appropriate music prerecorded for the workout activities. Make sure the audio equipment used has adequate sound quality. The music should be upbeat, contemporary, and most of all, motivating.

The fun begins with a couple of medium tempo songs to accompany warm-up exercises. The selection of songs may gradually introduce a slightly faster beat for aerobic games. Toward the end of the workout, the types of songs may gradually become slower in order to allow a cool down period.

There are many recordings which have inspired enthusiasm consistently. An example of such a song is <u>YMCA</u>. The children can create the Y-M-C-A with their bodies. They can even sing along and scream "YMCA" during the chorus.

Another great work out song is the <u>Theme From Rocky</u>. Almost everyone loves to pretend boxing. All of the children can stand in a circle and begin to box in the air.

A fun part of this work out could be when one child moves to the center of the circle and becomes the leader. All of the children must box in the same manner. Then another child takes the place of the leader, and demonstrates their own boxing style. This can be done throughout the entire song.

Once the upper body has been warmed-up, it becomes time to work on the mid-section. The musical selection may include many songs such as Twist And Shout, Peppermint Twist, and the original Twist. Now everyone is ready to start twisting away. The children can be taught to twist high, twist low, twist from one side of the room, and then to the other side.

Another fun game to play is the "Freeze Game". The children dance freestyle, and when the music stops, everyone will "freeze" in place. There are no rules applied to this game since the primary objective is give everyone a work out. If some children do not completely stop dancing when the music stops, they should still be allowed to continue dancing. At a *FIT-KID PARTY WORKOUT*, there are no losers. A variation of this game may have the children sit on the floor when the music stops. Children love participating in this game. Usually one to three songs is sufficient for this particular activity.

Another exciting game for the children is "Balloon-Up-Up-And-Away". A minimum of one balloon for each child is needed as well as some more up beat music. When the music begins, all of the children throw their balloon up in the air. Before the balloons touch the floor, each child must continue to hit their balloon to keep it afloat. This activity will stretch the entire body and is considered extremely beneficial to the cardiovascular system. The "Balloon-Up-Up-And-Away" may be played for about five minutes.

A game which I call "Jumping Balls" can be played for approximately ten minutes during fast, upbeat music. Five light weight rubber balls or NERF BALLS™ approximately the size of grapefruits will be needed. Additionally, an old or inexpensive sheet or tablecloth will be required. Cut a hole (slightly larger then the ball) in the center of the sheet. The sheet is then stretched out horizontally while the children hold the edges. Place the balls in the center. The object of the game is to have the children lift the sheet up and down until all five balls roll into the hole. This activity will strengthen the upper body.

Playing Limbo is always a favorite. All that is needed is Caribbean style music (Hot-Hot-Hot is a good choice for a song) and a stick (about four to five feet long). The game begins as the stick is placed high enough to allow all of the children to pass underneath. After the first pass, the stick is slightly lowered to increase the degree of difficulty. Each time, the stick gets a little lower. Unlike conventional Limbo, if a child touches the stick or cannot make it underneath, he or she is not out of the game. Instead, the child can hop over the stick. This change of rules will eliminate the chance that there may be children left on the sidelines. This game is over after everyone must hop over the stick.

Relay races are always fun at parties. It is extremely important to make sure that you have enough room for this activity. The relay race consist of at least two teams of equal numbers of children. About four upbeat songs can be used to motivate enthusiasm. The relay race can begin with each team balancing a hard-boiled egg on a spoon. The first child on each team will balance the egg while going toward a designated turning point. Once the child returns to the team, the next child in line can place a balloon between his or her legs while walking toward the same point. Once there, the child on each team can be instructed to hop back to their team.

There are many variations of the relay race. A hula hoop can be used as well as a small hard cover book (the children can improve their coordination by balancing the book on the head). The children will never get bored as long as there is a variety of activities. This game should last fifteen to twenty minutes. Always remember, everyone is a winner.

The children can be prepared for the cool down by using the party favorites <u>The Chicken Dance</u>, or the <u>Hokey-Pokey</u>. The children can create a circle. It is very important to have an adult participating in the entire workout. If the adult is at the same level with the children, the party will never get boring. When an adult becomes involved with the workout, it may be a good practice to exaggerate movements in front of the children. It may be necessary to become "larger than life" in order to gain a reaction.

Arrange to have the fitness game to last about forty-five minutes to an hour. This will allow enough time for eating and the distribution of presents and prizes without hurrying.

FIT-KID PARTY SAMPLE AGENDA

<u>A one-and-a-half to two hour party:</u>

<u>Activity</u>	<u>Amount of Time</u>
• Arrival of guests	15 minutes
• Fitness games	45 minutes to one hour
• Food and dessert	30 minutes
• Present opening (for a birthday)	20 minutes
• Distribute prizes, awards, trophies, and "goody-bags".	10 minutes

As all of the guests arrive sporadically, it is important to keep the children occupied which have already arrived. One idea which can be implemented easily is *edible jewelry*. Place a large blanket on the floor. Fill a large bowl with CHEERIOS™, and supply new thin shoe laces to the children. By tying a knot at the end of each lace, the children can create their own edible necklace. For older children, a large blunt needle and thread may used in order to string raisins, popcorn, and dried fruit.

How much could you expect to spend on a *FIT-KID PARTY*? Of course this depends largely on how lavish you want it to be. However, with a good plan, an entire *FIT-KID PARTY* held for twenty children (including invitations, decorations, food, paper goods, prizes, props, and thank you cards), can usually cost between two-hundred and two-hundred-and fifty dollars.

Remember, when planning a *FIT-KID PARTY*, keep the atmosphere fun and attitude upbeat. The key to a successful party is to keep the children moving from one activity to another smoothly - and have a fun *FIT-KID* time!

CHAPTER 7
WALL CHART OF SUCCESS

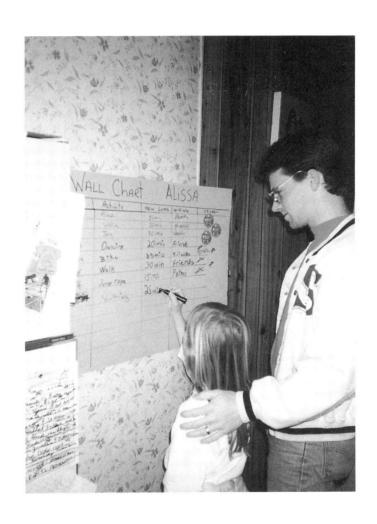

Seven

The Wall Chart of Success can be a valuable tool to help motivate children to exercise on a daily basis. Each day, children can fill in their chart and be rewarded with a success sticker. The success sticker can be placed on the wall chart at the end of every successful exercise day. If an activity was not completed for one particular day, a sticker would not be placed (this is why it's probably a good idea for the adults to apply the stickers).

The Wall Chart of Success can be made very easily. You will need a large piece of oak tag paper (any color), magic markers, and a large straight edge. I have provided a sample Wall Chart of Success in this chapter to be used as a model. The model is only a reference. You and the child can become creative by adding pictures (either pasted or drawn). A supply of success stickers will also be necessary. Allowing the child to select the which stickers he or she prefers is an excellent idea. The stickers can be purchased at a party store or almost any stationary store.

It will be necessary to make a new chart every month. Using the chart should be easy once the child becomes familiar with the details. You may want to explain to the child how the information is written onto the chart. This will in effect teach the child independence. For instance, the child will be responsible to enter the date, the type of activity, and in what length of time the activity was completed.

If one particular activity was accomplished everyday at the completion of one wall chart, the child can be rewarded with a small plastic trophy. This type of reward will provide an added incentive to work toward. These type of trophies can be purchased at a party store for approximately two dollars (well worth the investment).

Most children love others to watch their progress. It's a good idea to place the wall chart in a visible part of the house (possibly the kitchen). This in turn makes a child feel very important.

Wall Chart of Success

NAME:			AGE:	
Day / Date	**Type Of Activity**	**How long did activity last ?**	**How far did you go ?**	**Success Sticker**
Tues/ February 2	Jogging	30 min.	2 times around the block	✕
Weds./ February 3	Walking with Mommy	30 min.	Half-Mile	✕

CHAPTER 8
PRAISE FOR PLAY

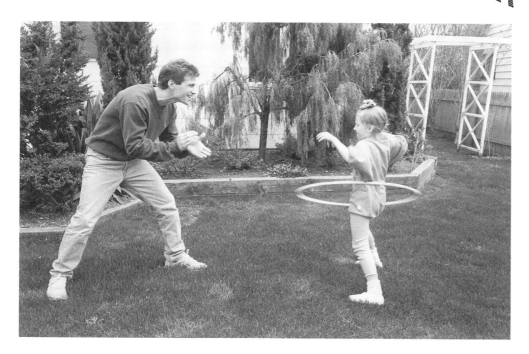

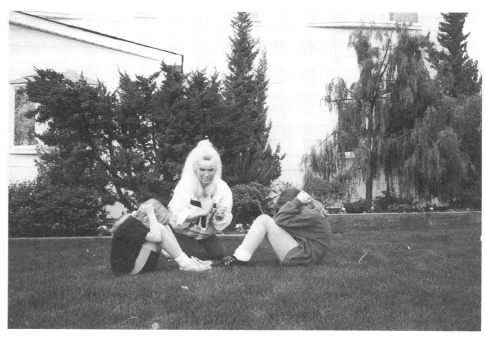

Eight

What is motivation? Motivation has been defined as a provided need or desire which causes a person to act. Essentially, motivation may be referred to as an inner drive stimulated by an incentive. When discussing children and exercise, *fun* should always be the primary motivation.

Motivation stimulates action. Motivation is not permanent, but neither is eating or exercise. In order to instill a positive attitude within the child, a certain amount of motivation and praise must be applied on a daily basis.

A negative attitude can be the most destructive force that can affect a child. To tell a child that he or she "is no good", "can't do that", or "will never amount to anything", can produce damaging results that can last throughout life. Any sense of confidence is basically stripped away from the child.

Anyone who comes in contact with a child must offer hope, encouragement, and belief. This practice should be continuous and sincere. Encouragement should be given to the child regardless of the magnitude of the accomplishment. The benefits of praise will define the entire lifestyle of the child. It may become most noticeable in the type and regularity of exercises.

All children require (and constantly look for) praise and attention from parents, teachers, and peers. Praise can be given for any reason in terms such as "I'm so proud of you", "excellent job", and "way to go". By being exposed to similar examples of encouragement, a child will quickly achieve a greater sense of confidence and self-esteem.

In the home, parents should create an atmosphere which will encourage a child to participate in physical activity. However, setting the stage for exercise and sports related activities should always be done without inducing pressure on the child. Allow children to be children. Exploring and creating is a large part of growing up. The objective is to have the child become involved with activity, not try to create an Olympic athlete. The goal of parents is to promote a fun, healthy attitude toward fitness and nutrition.

Many times, a negative approach is used when trying to motivate a child to exercise. A child should not be told of statistics involving children with poor health such as heart attacks. Additionally, the terms "you'll get fat if you don't exercise" and "couch potato" should never be used. Moreover, exercise must not be turned into a "have-to-do" project. Force never becomes fun. Instead, only rejection will result.

A child should never be *bribed* to exercise with a toy or special food treat. The child will not develop the belief that exercise in itself is beneficial when this particular type of reward behavior is used.

Alternative methods of initiating incentives which may be used are a *Fitness Progress Record-Keeping System* and *Motivation Star Stickers*. The *Fitness Progress Record-Keeping System* is discussed in detail in chapter seven, Wall Chart Of Success.

Motivation Star Stickers can be given to the child as a reward without becoming pretentious. A variety of stickers which depict animated characters and designs can be used to eliminate the factor of predictability.

It is very important to never compare the accomplishments of one child to another. If any comparison is made, have the child only compare their most recent progression of an activity to the previous achievement. Participation, not competition is the key.

THINGS TO REMEMBER

- In order to instill a positive attitude to create a happy, healthy child, the adult (parent, teacher, etc.) must be positive and happy. Positive feedback such as "I'm proud of you", "you did great", and " excellent job" will always produce positive results.
- In terms of the fitness and progress of the child, always look at the glass as half-full, never half-empty.
- Using the philosophy "you are what you think you are", tell the child that he or she is the best. If you believe in the abilities of the child (and everything they do), the child will also.
- The way in which someone thinks, is probably how they will perform. If as a role model, you can display a genuine acceptance of exercising, the child too will become receptive to exercise.
- A smile given freely from a parent to a child is an excellent, non-verbal expression of reinforcement and love.
- Applause is the most valuable encouragement a child can receive.

THINGS TO REMEMBER (continued)

- In the vocabulary of a child, leave the "T" out of "CAN'T".

- Always keep the lines of communication open with a child. A child should not be afraid to be honest about any subject.

- Always let the child know that you understand, and are always available for him or her.

- Children must be taught to concentrate on what they can do and improve on that one particular activity. Children should not spend any time concentrating, and inevitably, worrying about things they cannot do.

Always discover the best within a child and applaud the results. There are millions of parents who love their children. But very often, the love and encouragement is not expressed with applause. Applauding can build confidence quickly, which in turn, raises the progressive growth of the child physically, mentally, and emotionally. Children, in general, require a constant reminder that they did well.

Affirmation is a tool for helping children succeed. Affirmation assumes the form of a positive thought, which can take the place of a negative thought. Eventually, positive focusing can become inherent.

It is possible that the single most important thing children can receive from a parent, teacher, or another role model, is belief in themselves. High self-esteem is a major ingredient of success. Very often, high self-esteem begins with childhood experiences.

If a child becomes involved in an exercise plan or fitness routine, it is an absolute necessity to remember all of the suggestions mentioned within this chapter. Praise and encouragement must be given to the *FIT-KID* on a daily basis.

CHAPTER 9
REWARDING THE FITNESS PROCESS

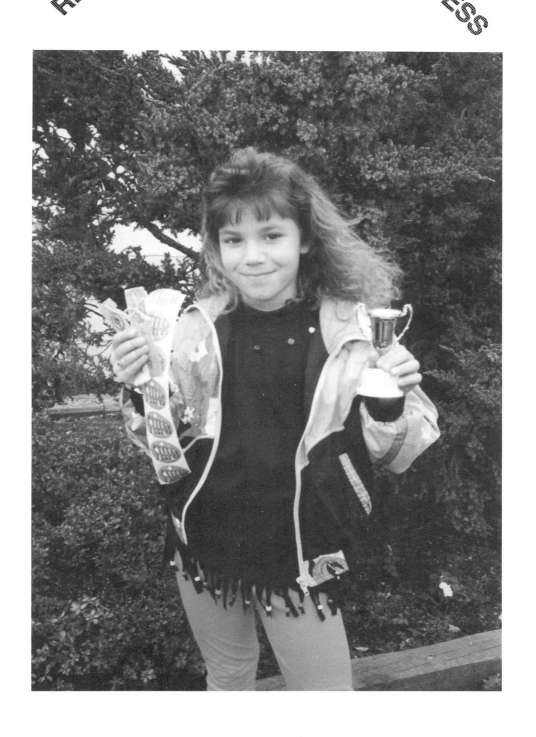

Nine

How do you get kids off the couch and into exercising? The same way you get them to do almost anything - bribery. Actually, that statement is slightly facetious. The truth is that most adults use food as a reward when attempting to get a child to do anything. This is the last thing that a sedentary or overweight child needs.

There are many less fattening reinforcements to encourage a child to get up and begin moving. This can be achieved by rewarding the process of fitness as well as the final results.

Rewarding children after the completion of an exercise activity is an added incentive which can enhance pride and excitement. Rewards that a child receive can be based on completing an activity on a daily basis initially. The reward can then graduate to weekly, and eventually, monthly.

A reward that is given to a child should not be food, toys, or clothes. Instead, awards which represent achievement such as *success stickers, ribbons,* and *trophies* can be used as exceptional motivating tools. A variety of stickers, ribbons, and trophies can be purchased inexpensively at a party supply store or stationary store.

Stickers have been found to be a favorite among children. Gold star stickers are especially significant when they are used to represent an award. However, it is very important to allow the child to select a favorite sticker. The stickers can be used as a daily reward for a "job well done" in conjunction with an exercise activity.

It is not necessary for a child to finish in first place during a race in order to receive a ribbon and feel special. A ribbon can be given to child after the completion of a week's worth of activities. For instance, if a child collects seven stickers, he or she will be entitled to a ribbon.

Most children love to receive trophies as an award. A trophy can be a very effective tool in raising self esteem within a child. This type of reward should be given on a monthly basis when a child accomplishes a series of activities when he or she has collected four ribbons.

If a child has missed a day of activities, he or she should not be scolded. With the reward system and variety of incentives outlined in this chapter, the child should be encouraged to pursue even a simple activity. If this is not possible, reassurance that tomorrow is another day would probably be the best approach.

Encouraging a child to participate in a activity every day will begin a practice which will most probably be carried into adulthood. As the child matures, the distribution of *success stickers, ribbons,* and *trophies* will dissipate. However, the rewards realized will be in the form of overall better health, more energy, and a greater feeling of self-confidence.

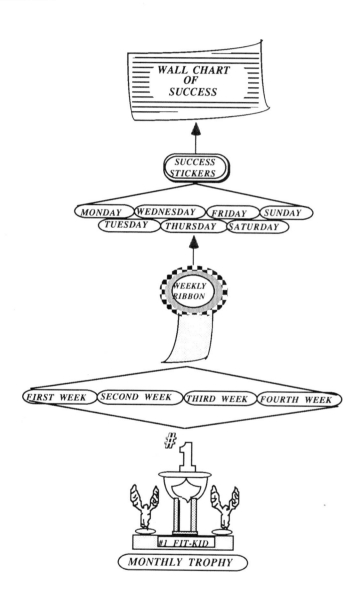

FIT-KIDS: GETTING KIDS "HOOKED" ON FITNESS FUN!

CHAPTER 10
ROLE MODELS

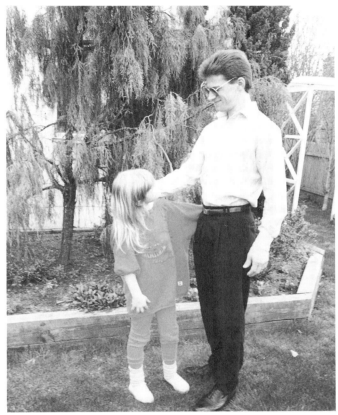

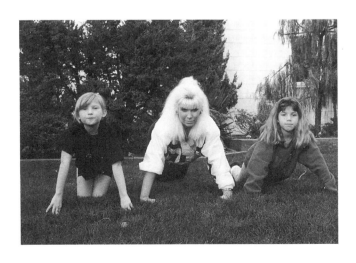

Ten

There are going to be many influential individuals in a child's life. Some of these people will be considered role models. In most cases, parents and teachers will affect a child in this manner.

A role model should have positive personality traits. I have listed several important qualities which a *role model* should possess.

<u>Positive attitude</u> - a person with a positive attitude refuses to dwell on anything negative. This type of person will seek positive aspects from every situation.

<u>Enthusiasm</u> - anything that an enthusiastic person becomes involved with is very important. A person with a great deal of enthusiasm will give one-hundred and twenty percent of effort, all of the time.

<u>Persistence</u> - a persistent person will never quit out of frustration or other negative influences. Persistence will lead a person to complete anything in which they set out to do.

<u>Patience</u> - the capacity to deal with imperfection without assigning fault requires patience. Anyone who pursues a multitude of activities must become patient with their own progress. When such an attitude is displayed, children will quickly grasp the usefulness of patience.

If parents are to set examples as role models, it may be necessary to reinforce several guidelines. The guidelines listed below may not be easy to follow at first. However, as with any new behavior patterns, it will just require a little time to realize the benefits.

1. <u>BEHAVIOR</u> - Parents should maintain a calm, even temperament. When parents begin to raise their voices and display vulgarity at small disturbances, children will begin to adopt these behavior patterns as their own.

2. <u>EXERCISE</u> - If parents maintain an exercise program, credibility is established more readily when trying to instill these values to children.

3. <u>FUN</u> - Parents should always emphasize fitness as fun. The best image for the parent to project to the child is that exercise and good nutrition is fun and interesting, not difficult or comparable with a chore. If a parent displays excessive aches and pains as well as *huffing and puffing* after a workout, it is very likely that the child will be hesitant to become involved in exercise. On the contrary, a child will be quickly attracted to fitness if they see a parent say something similar to *"I feel great, I have so much energy"*.

4. NO SMOKING - At the very least, cigarette smoking should be eliminated from the home. It is no secret that cigarette smoking has been linked to heart disease and cancer. But if this hasn't been an incentive to stop, then preventing to set a terrible example for children should be the motivating factor. If mom and dad smoke, it is very likely that the children will assume the habit is acceptable.

5. LIMITED T.V. VIEWING - If a television curfew has not yet been set within a household, it may be necessary to implement one. By reducing the amount of time a child will watch television on a daily basis will increase the possibility of pursuing an exercise program.

6. NUTRITION - All bad eating habits are learned. You are not born with them. Food is administered to stop an infant from crying. Food is given to a toddler as a reward for "being good" or simply for an accomplishment. As a child matures, he or she is told to "finish everything on the plate so you can have dessert". These examples are early beginnings to poor eating habits that could possibly follow a child into adulthood.

Children can easily develop the taste for sweets and fatty foods just like their parents because they haven't been exposed to any other way of eating. If parents set examples of eating healthy (fruit, pretzels, and baked foods instead of candy, potato chips, and fried foods respectively), children would be sure to follow.

This part of being a role model is arguably the most important. The following chapters in this book address the subject of nutrition;

Creating a healthy role model for children is an absolute necessity. By successfully achieving this goal, children will be rewarded with a head start toward a healthy adulthood.

CHAPTER 11
FAT-PROOFING YOUR HOME

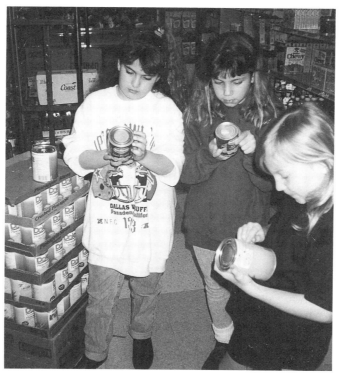

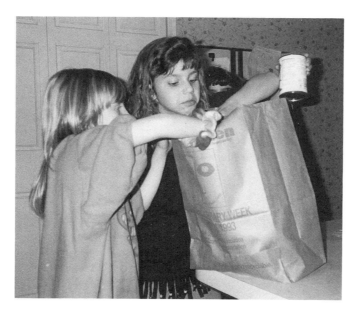

Eleven

Proper nutrition is vitally important to the health of a child. All food habits are learned by early experiences with food. Proper nutrition begins at home. Parents are instrumental in the learning process of a child regarding proper nutrition. A parent can easily begin to guide the eating habits of a child by setting a good example.

Unfortunately, there is much room for improvement when discussing the eating habits of families in America. Presently, there are millions of obese children in this country. Most of the children will carry their obesity into adulthood. The majority of which will suffer unhappy physical, social, and psychological consequences throughout their life.

Throughout my years of research, most overweight children have at least one parent who is also overweight. Apparently, the children grow up within an environment in which a role model (parent) has a propensity toward over eating.

A person of this nature may believe that food exists to produce pure gratification. This type of behavior pattern is then imitated by the children of such parents. The overweight family lives to eat, they don't eat to live.

91

Weight control and proper nutrition must be established early in life. By the time a child reaches three years of age, he or she may be easily influenced by outside sources.

Television plays one of the biggest roles in regard to influencing children. Children spend an average of three hours a day viewing television. During this time, the children are being slowly convinced by advertisers that sugar sweetened cereals are good for them. Most of the cereals targeted toward children include a prize as an added incentive.

For the most part, children do not comprehend nutrition without guidance. It is difficult for a child to understand that many foods advertised on television may not be the best choice. Nor does the child realize the consequences which may occur later in life (such as heart disease and obesity).

It is very important to expose children to the four food groups. I call it the *FAB FOUR*. A child will become more receptive to this information if it has a *cool* name. Basic nutrition should be learned at an early age in order for children to develop proper eating habits which will last a lifetime. Moreover, if a child is to effectively learn about nutrition, he or she must have fun. *Kids* , for the most part, will only do things that look like it may be fun and enjoyable.

Most children are not in need of a strict diet. But like most adults, children must replace old eating habits with healthy new habits. In order to get a child involved with the healthy food concept, the following guidelines may be used;

1. Educate the child (children) about the *FAB FOUR*, and reading food labels.

2. Create the food shopping list with the entire family.

92

3. Make food shopping a family event.

4. Enlist the assistance of the child when preparing and cooking the meal.

5. Have the child (children) help set the table.

All of the guidelines mentioned will establish the child as an integral part of meal planning and preparation (as well as learning to become more independent). In addition to spending quality time with Mom and Dad, having a child participate in the entire nutrition process will enable him or her to acquire valuable knowledge.

Before you can begin *Fat-proofing* your home, the basic four food groups must be reviewed. Along with this activity, reading food labels and learning about various ingredients will become a common practice.

In order to obtain the proper nutrients, it is important to eat a variety of foods from the four food groups on a daily basis. The *FAB FOUR* food groups are as follows;

1. DAIRY - good for bones and teeth.

2. BREAD / CEREAL - good source of energy.

3. MEAT / PROTEIN - good for building and repairing muscles.

4. FRUITS / VEGETABLES - good for eyes and skin.

Some of the foods which do not belong to the *FAB FOUR* food groups are as follows;

A. FATS - such as butter and mayonnaise.

B. SWEETS - such as jellies, sodas, candies.

C. SALT

I have created *FIT-KID FUN ACTIVITIES* which you and a child can use to evaluate proper nutrition. Since children love to do these activities more than once, it may be a good idea to create copies of the following pages. Additionally, the lessons of proper nutrition will be reinforced by repeating the written exercises.

THE FOUR FOOD GROUPS

ACTIVITY #1

Have the child write the names of three foods in each of the four groups.

FRUITS & VEGETABLES

1. _____
2. _____
3. _____

MEAT & PROTEIN FOODS

1. _____
2. _____
3. _____

BREAD & GRAINS

1. _____
2. _____
3. _____

DAIRY FOODS

1. _____
2. _____
3. _____

ACTIVITY #2

Have the child cross-out the food which does not belong in each of the blocks, then write the name of the food group.

MUFFIN	CEREAL
CARROT	BREAD

_____ GROUP

EGG	CHEESE
CHICKEN	CANDY

_____ GROUP

YOGURT	ICE CREAM
MILK	COOKIES

_____ GROUP

EGG	GRAPES
APPLE	BANANA

_____ GROUP

ACTIVITY #3

Many foods are made up of more than one food group. This activity will teach a child how to identify each item of food.

By using the guideline provided (see below), see if a child could identify each food group in the foods illustrated by inserting the proper number in the circle.

GUIDELINE

1. FRUITS / VEGETABLES

2. MEAT / PROTEIN

3. BREAD / GRAINS

4. DAIRY

broccoli
cake
pork chop
strawberry
potato
hamburger
yogurt
carrot

cheese
french fries
rye bread
ice cream
bagel
cupcake
chicken
popcorn

EXAMPLE

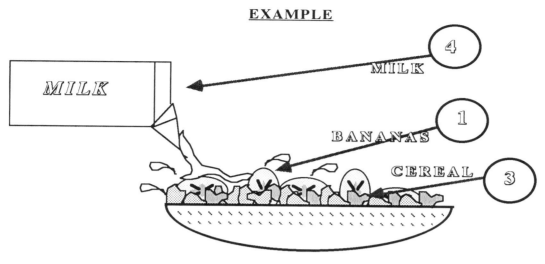

FILL IN THE CORRECT FOOD GROUP NUMBERS
TO IDENTIFY EACH
FOOD ITEM SHOWN.

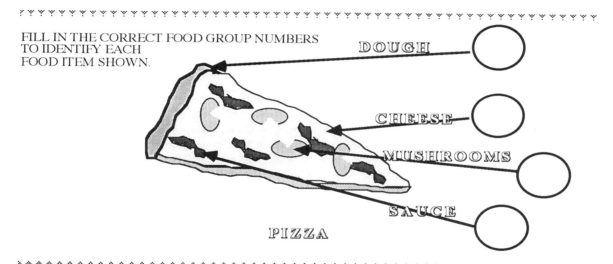

FILL IN THE CORRECT FOOD GROUP NUMBERS
TO IDENTIFY EACH
FOOD ITEM SHOWN.

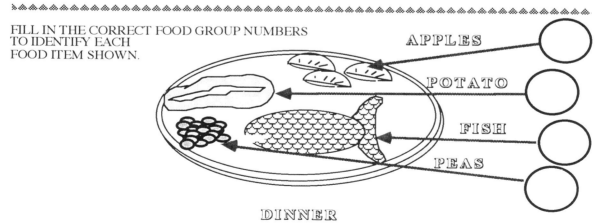

ACTIVITY #4

This particular activity is simply called *WRITE IT DOWN*. By maintaining a food diary for a one week period, it's easy to see if the basic nutrition requirements are being met.

An adult and child can participate in this activity together by writing down everything that is consumed during the course of the day. It could be interesting to see if certain goals of meeting the requirements of the four food groups are reached each day.

In order to enhance this activity, each food group may be highlighted with a separate color marker. For example:

YELLOW for Dairy

RED for Fruits & Vegetables

BLUE for Bread & Grains

PINK for Meat & Protein

ACTIVITY #5

Let's call this activity "IT'S IN THE BAG". Give a child a brown paper lunch bag. A drawing of a bag can be used as well (copy the bag illustrated on the following page). Have the child cut out foods which represent the four food groups from a magazine or supermarket circular (at least one item from each group). Each item found can be glued or taped onto the bag.

NOTE: It's extremely important to check the selections the child makes, and to make any corrections necessary.

"IT'S IN THE BAG"

DON'T FORGET US !

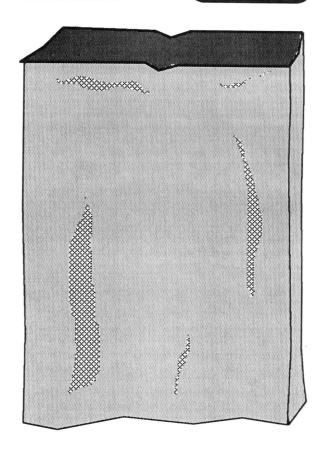

DAIRY FOODS

BREAD & CEREAL GRAINS

MEAT & PROTEIN FOODS

FRUITS & VEGETABLES

SERVING SIZES FOR CHILDREN

BREAD GROUP

Children require **six servings** of food from this group everyday. Bread and grain help supply the child with energy to think and play.

FRUIT AND VEGETABLE GROUP

A child requires at least **three servings** of food from the vegetable group and at least **two servings** of fruit everyday. Fruit and vegetables gives the body the vitamins required for healthy skin, hair, and eyes.

DAIRY GROUP

A child requires a minimum of **three servings** from the dairy group everyday. The dairy group gives the body strong bones and teeth.

MEAT AND PROTEIN GROUP

It is important for a child to acquire at least **two servings** from the meat and protein group on a daily basis. This group will help the body grow.

LEARNING "HOW TO READ" FOOD LABELS

It is very important to select foods which have the largest nutritional value. But sometimes it's difficult to tell how nutritious a particular food is just by looking at it. This is why *NUTRITION LABELING* is so important. This type of labeling is presently available on almost all purchased food. Below is an example of a typical nutrition label.

PRODUCT: RAISIN FLAKES (high fiber cereal)

Serving Size: **2/3 cup**   Servings per container: **7**

	Cereal	**Skim milk**
Calories	120	160
Protein	3 g	7 g
Carbohydrate	31 g	37 g
Fat	1 g	0 g
Cholesterol	0 g	260 g
Sodium	200 g	260 g
Potassium	260 g	460 g

Percentages of U.S. Recommended Daily Allowances (USRDA)

	Cereal	**Skim milk**
Protein	41%	10%
Vitamin A	35%	40%
Vitamin C	-----	2%
Thiamine	35%	40%
Iron	35%	35%
Folic acid	35%	35%
Vitamin B 6	35%	35%
Vitamin B 12	35%	35%
Zinc	15%	20%
Copper	10%	20%

INGREDIENTS: Whole wheat, raisins, sugar, natural flavoring, corn syrup, honey.

SERVING INFORMATION

Nutritional information is based on each serving. It is important to know how large one serving is (example; 1/2 cup, 2 ounces, 1 slice).

The next piece of information to look for is the number of servings each package or can contains. For instance, if the serving size on a label is two ounces, and the package contains a total of eight ounces, there are four servings of that product in that particular container.

There are sections of the nutrition label which detail the amount of calories, protein carbohydrates, and fat in each serving of the product. This information is presented in grams, which is represented by a "g". If a label states "Protein ...2g", there are two grams of protein in one serving of that particular product. For a simple conversion from grams to ounces, there are twenty-eight grams in one ounce.

The section of a food label that is called *Percentage of U.S. Recommended Daily Allowances* (U.S.R.D.A.) will illustrate a portion (shown as a percentage) of various vitamins and minerals. The U.S.R.D.A. should be used as guide. The type and amount of food consumed should provide one-hundred percent (or reasonably close) of the vitamins and minerals necessary on a daily basis.

Within the U.S.R.D.A. section of a nutrition label, at least five vitamins should be listed as well as calcium and iron. Foods which do not contain all vitamins and minerals, the list will state that the product contains less than two percent of the U.S.R.D.A. of vitamin A, thiamine, and calcium. Additionally, some labels will list cholesterol and sodium for people who must maintain restricted diets.

DEFINITIONS

CALORIE

A calorie is a measure of heat energy needed to raise the temperature of one liter of water one degree centigrade. Calories in food become energy to our bodies. Similar to gasoline in a car, a car cannot operate without gas. Our bodies cannot run on empty without food.

The amount of calories needed depends on your age, and the amount of activities you do. If a person takes in more calories than their body requires, the calories will be stored as fat.

PROTEIN

Protein builds and repairs cells. Additionally, protein also helps fight infections and makes blood strong. Some excellent sources of protein can be found in fish, meat, eggs, and milk.

CARBOHYDRATES

Carbohydrates provide energy for muscles, nerves and the brain.

Complex carbohydrates provide calories and other nutrients which are essential for digestion and prevention of some diseases. *Complex carbohydrates* are also considered to be a great source of fiber. A good source of *Complex carbohydrates* can be found in bread, noodles, grain, potatoes, nuts, peas, and fruit.

Simple carbohydrates provide calories, but not much of anything else. *Simple carbohydrates* will give a fast rise in blood sugar for a surge of energy. Sources of *Simple carbohydrates* can be found in sugar and honey.

FAT

Fat provides energy and helps digestion. However, too much fat can be harmful. A good source of fat can be found in vegetable oils, butter, cheeses, eggs, chocolate, and peanut butter.

VITAMINS

Vitamins help the body use food and work properly. Vitamins are found in each of the four food groups. Especially good sources of vitamins are carrots, lettuce, cantaloupe, milk, fish, poultry, and meat. It may be a good idea to supplement a diet (especially the diet of a child) with multi-vitamins. There are a variety of excellent multivitamins which offer attractive boxes, shapes, and appealing tastes.

MINERALS

Minerals strengthen bones, teeth, and blood. Minerals also help the body use energy. Calcium is found within the dairy group. Iron can be found in liver, kidney, peas, and dark green leafy vegetables.

WATER

More than half of a persons body weight is attributed to water. Without water, the body would become dehydrated very quickly. Water transports nutrients to cells and assists in the disposal of waste. Additionally, water aids in digestion and regulates body temperature.

It is strongly recommended that a person consume eight glasses of water daily. A good source of water can be found in fruit juices and other beverages.

SUGAR

Did you know the average person consumes 125 pounds of sugar in one year? Children should become aware of the various names that sugar is referred to as in the ingredient listings;

SUGAR
BROWN SUGAR
RAW SUGAR
HONEY
MAPLE SYRUP
CORN SYRUP
HIGH FRUCTOSE
CORN SWEETENER
SUCROSE
FRUCTOSE
LACTOSE
MALT

A good activity to learn about sugar is to have children collect various boxes of cereal, cookies, snacks, etc. Have each child look for the names which identify the ingredient as sugar (using the list above). Then, have child circle all of the different names.

105

GET KIDS "HOOKED" ON NATURE'S CANDY...FRUIT

Ask children to name their favorite sweet snack or dessert. In most cases, children will reply with the answer "cookies", "candy", or "ice cream". Then ask the children "Do you know what it is about fruit that is similar to the snacks they chose?" You can tell the children that fruit has a sweet taste (just like candy) because of the sugar content. The only difference is that fresh fruit has a much lower calorie count.

Children may become slightly confused at this premise and reply with "Isn't sugar, sugar?". The difference between candy (or another type of sweet snack) and fresh fruit can be easily explained. Processed sweet snacks often contain a large amount of sugar and fat, and very little in the way of vitamins, minerals, starch, and fiber. Sweet fruits contain some sugar, and next to no fat.

"FINDING OUT ALL THE FATS"

Children should learn about the various types of "fats". It's important to tell kids that it is a good idea to cut back on all kinds of fat. However, certain fats are more helpful than others.

The less harmful fats are <u>unsaturated fats</u>. This type of fat originates in vegetables and fish. the unsaturated fats stay in liquid form. Olive oil is a good example of an unsaturated fat.

<u>Saturated fats</u> most often originate from animals (meat, poultry, dairy products). These fats are typically solid at room temperature. Butter is a good example of a saturated fat.

Cholesterol is a fatty substance found in animal fats. Egg yolks have a large content of fat and cholesterol. It is extremely important to teach children that saturated fat and cholesterol in food raise the cholesterol content in the body. An excessive amount of cholesterol can build up within the arteries of the body, and eventually "clog" or close them. This, of course, adds an increased risk for heart disease, obesity, and high blood pressure.

Teaching children to eat food which is low in fat can be achieved by explaining how to read food labels. By exercising this practice, a child can learn to select foods which are low in fat and cholesterol.

FOOD LABELING REFORMS

To further inform consumers about the nutritional content of the foods they select, the Federal Food and Drug Administration will be issuing new regulations for food manufacturers. These new regulations will include "mandatory and consistent" nutrition labels.

The new nutrition labels are to include the following:

• Amounts of saturated fat, fiber, cholesterol, and calories from fat.

• Definitions of food descriptions and claims such as "low fat", "high fiber", and "low cholesterol".

• Standardizing serving sizes to make food comparisons more exact.

EXAMPLE OF THE NEW NUTRITION LABEL

PRODUCT: RICE

Nutrition Information Per Serving

Serving Size...............................45 grams (about 1 cup cooked)

Servings per container..................30

Calories..160

Calories from fat..............................4

Total fat..*

Saturated...*

Unsaturated..*

Total carbohydrate........................35 grams

Complex carbohydrates................34 grams

Sugars..*

Dietary fiber.......................................*

Protein..4 grams

Sodium...0 grams

* MEANS LESS THAN 1 GRAM

By the end of 1993, the majority of food products will have the updated nutrition label. Since some products may remain equipped with the original label, it is important for a child to be able to read and understand both.

INGREDIENTS ON A LABEL

Labels on food products list ingredients in a descending order (from the most to the least). A good math and nutrition activity may be the collection of food labels, then ask the following questions:

1) How many ingredients does each product have?
2) Which ingredient is most abundant?
3) Which ingredient is least abundant?

Food selections based on nutrition labeling can make a terrific show and tell project at home or school. The object of this activity is the detection of foods which are high in fat, calories, and sugar.

Have a child (or group of children) peel off labels from cans and cut out labels from boxes. Then, tell the child (or children) that he or she is going to become the *LABEL DETECTIVE* .

With the labels available, have the children create four categories; high fat, high calories, high sugar, and healthy food. The job of the child is to identify the food label as one of the four categories, then place it into that particular section. The healthy food category would include food labels which are low in fat, calories, and sugar.

It may be necessary to check the results of the activity. The accuracy of identifying the food labels is essential to the child becoming correctly informed.

BUILDING A HEALTHY SANDWICH

What does it take to build a healthy sandwich? It can probably be compared to building a house. First, you will need a good foundation. You should then be well equipped with the building materials. This may be followed by one or several additions.

There are items listed below which are divided into three categories, *FOUNDATIONS, BUILDING MATERIALS,* and *ADDITIONS* . Have a child select an item from each category in order to build a healthy sandwich.

FOUNDATIONS	*BUILDING MATERIALS*	*ADDITIONS*
White bread	Chicken	Mayonnaise
Roll	Cheese	Butter
Bagel	Hard Boiled Egg	Plain yogurt
Pita Bread	Cottage Cheese	Nuts
Crackers	Turkey	Mustard
Whole Wheat Bread	Fish	Catsup
Taco Shell	Beef	Lettuce
Corn muffin		Tomatoes

MAKE A PERFECT SALAD

Have a child turn into a "make-believe" chef and circle several of the ingredients listed below in order to create a perfect salad (be careful of the ingredients that don't belong in a healthy salad).

TOMATOES   RADISHES

LITE SALAD DRESSING

LETTUCE   NUTS

CUCUMBER

RED CABBAGE   RAISIN

BROCCOLI

MUSHROOM   COOKIES

POTATOES

PEAS   ZUCCHINI

MUFFIN

CANDY   ONIONS

ICE CREAM

MELON   CROUTONS

JELLY

OIL & VINEGAR DRESSING

HEALTHY FOODS & ACTIVITIES vs. HEALTH-HURTERS

Making kids aware of what are healthy foods and activities as opposed to "health-hurters" early in life will help them develop positive, healthy lifestyles.

Identifying the "health- hurters" before adulthood is essential in order to avoid chronic health problems. Listed below in random are healthy foods and activities as well as "health-hurters". Have a child circle all items which represent a healthy lifestyle, and cross-out the "health-hurters".

DAILY EXERCISE   HIGH SUGAR FOODS

                 SMOKING

SKIPPING BREAKFAST   SALADS

                 POPCORN

FRIED FOODS   SANDWICHES

           TOO MUCH T.V.

COOKIES   BACON

                CANDY

YOGURT   FATTY FOODS

Using the items listed below, have a child cross out any food which includes "processed sugar" in the ingredients. **HELPFUL HINT:** Create photocopies of this list in order to repeat this activity in the future.

COTTON CANDY

ORANGE JUICE

BANANA

ICE CREAM

RAISIN

COOKIES

MUFFIN

MELON

PEAR

APPLE PIE

GRAPES

ORANGE

MUSHROOM

PEAS

CANDY

JELLY

NUTRITION FLASH CARDS

Most children love to make math and reading flash cards out of ordinary index cards. With this activity, we can create nutrition fun into flash card fun.

You will need the following items for this activity;

1) About twenty to thirty index cards (any size).

2) Marker pen

3) Transparent tape / glue.

4) Various pictures of food (can be cut-out from magazines, circulars, etc.).

Half of the fun of this activity is actually making the cards. Secure the pictures of the food onto separate index cards with transparent tape or glue (if the children involved are older, pictures can be substituted with just the name of the food). Depending on the types of food chosen, categorize each food by writing onto the back of each card the following information;

1) Type of food group.

2) Nutritious food or a "junk food".

3) High in sugar?

4) High in fat?

This activity really sharpens nutrition skills, and kids love it!

114

AIMING FOR PROPER NUTRITION

Fun games for kids while learning the differences between fatty foods, high processed sugar foods, and healthy foods.

Material that will be needed for this activity;

1) Three coffee cans or shoe boxes.

2) Paper.

3) Crayons.

4) Scissors.

5) Pictures of food (taken from magazines or circulars).

6) Six bean bags or ping-pong balls).

Have the child decorate each one the containers to depict similar designs as illustrated below;

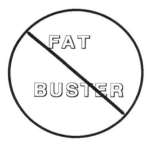 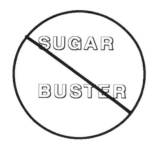 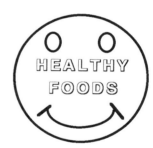

Use the pictures of food (or the nutrition flash cards created earlier in this chapter). Someone will be designated to show the picture (or card) to the child or children. Have the child stand approximately four feet from the empty containers. The child will decide which one of the three containers to throw the bean bag or ping-pong ball into.

This activity also helps eye-hand coordination!

TURNING "HEALTH-HURTERS" INTO HEALTHY FOODS

Have a child draw a line from the food listed in the left column to the compatible healthy food in the right column.

"HEALTH-HURTERS"	"HEALTHY FOODS"
FRIED CHICKEN	BAKED FISH
FRENCH FRIES	BAKED POTATO
APPLE PIE	BAKED CHICKEN
FRIED FISH	BAKED APPLE with cinnamon

MOVIE FOOD NUTRITION

When children go to the movies or watch a video at home, what types of food do they eat? Have the child circle each food listed below that are considered healthy snacks, perfect for movie viewing.

POPCORN (without butter)	COOKIES
CANDY	GRAPES
YOGURT	BANANA
ICE CREAM	ORANGE
RAISIN	SODA
GRAPE JUICE	SLICED APPLE

REWARDING THE NUTRITION "HABIT"

Just like the rewards which are given for exercise accomplishments, it is as important to reward eating healthy and learning about positive nutrition.

The following page illustrates a certificate. Make copies of it, write the name of the child into the area which is left blank (following the statement "THIS CERTIFIES THAT..."), then hang it up in a prominent location for all family members and friends to see.

IN A NUTSHELL

Children and adults alike must get into the habit of...

- increasing the consumption of fresh fruit and vegetables

- decreasing the consumption of refined and other processed sugar (cut-out candy, cakes, etc.)

- decreasing the consumption of foods high in fat (fried foods, oils) -replace with broiled and baked foods.

Eating healthy is a learned skill. Parents and children alike must learn healthy eating habits. Together, everyone will discover how to live happy and healthy lives.

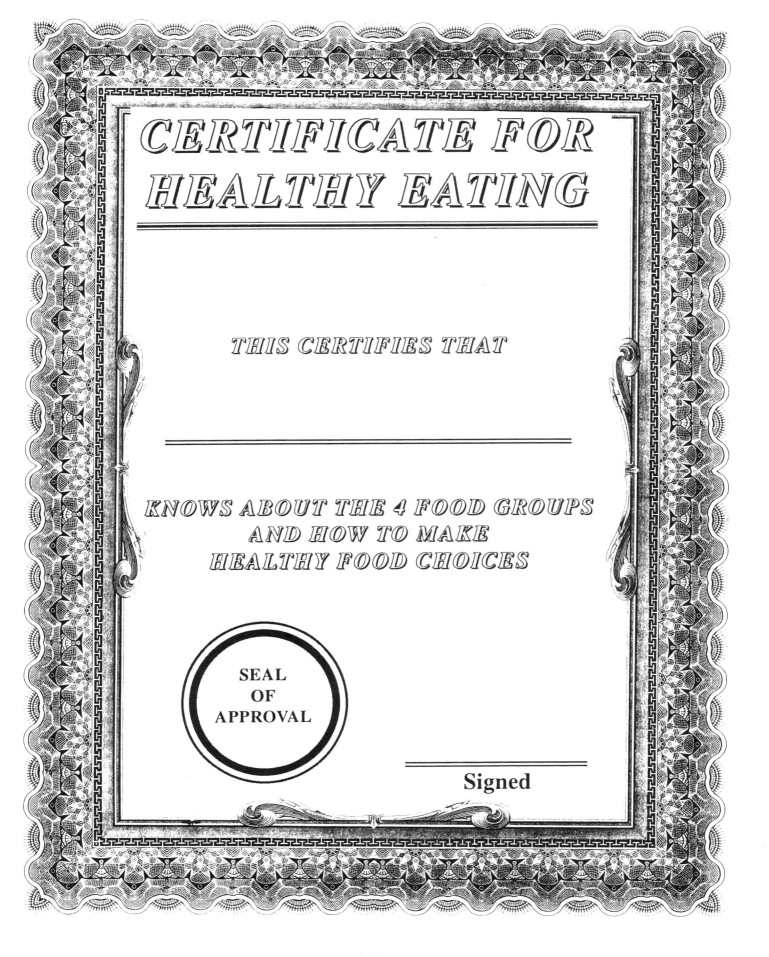

CERTIFICATE FOR HEALTHY EATING

THIS CERTIFIES THAT

KNOWS ABOUT THE 4 FOOD GROUPS AND HOW TO MAKE HEALTHY FOOD CHOICES

SEAL
OF
APPROVAL

Signed

FIT-KIDS: GETTING KIDS "HOOKED" ON FITNESS FUN!

CHAPTER 12

FOOD-SHOPPING WITH THE KIDS

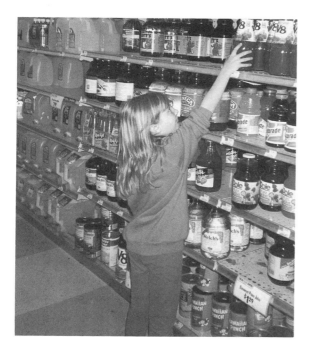

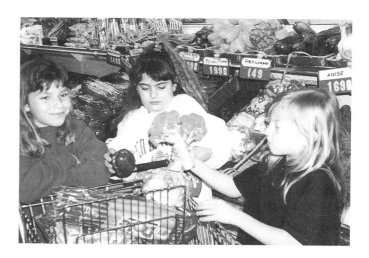

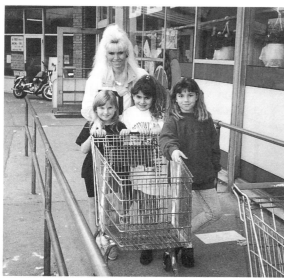

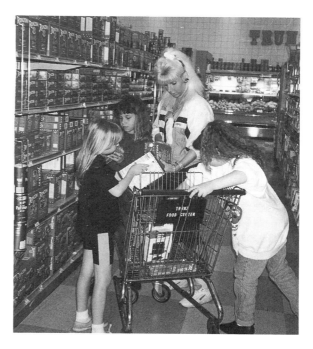

Twelve

Supermarket shopping can be a very educational and fun experience for a child. It can create a feeling of importance and arouse their interest in different types of food. A child can be made to feel as if he or she has control over what they choose.

A child that is allowed to select part of the daily menu is more likely to be cooperative about eating. The following food shopping related tasks can be shared;

- Making the food shopping list.
- Picking the products off the supermarket shelves and placing them into a shopping cart.
- Placing the products from the shopping cart onto the checkout counter.
- Unpacking and storing the food at home.

These activities will make children become excited and knowledgeable about various foods (before sharing the supermarket experience with your child, be sure to read chapter eleven, Fat-proofing Your Home).

PREPARING THE SHOPPING LIST WITH YOUR CHILD

Prepare a sheet of paper into sections with the name of a particular food group as the heading. Ask your child to help decide which food should be purchased. There is a sample of the shopping list below.

FRESH FRUITS

APPLES
CANTELOPE
ORANGES

FRESH VEGETABLES

CORN
LETTUCE
POTATO

DAIRY FOODS

SKIM MILK
COTTAGE CHEESE
YOGURT

BREADS / CEREALS

WHEAT BREAD
CORN FLAKES
PITA BREAD

MEATS / PROTEINS

CHICKEN
FISH
EGGS

BEVERAGES

ORANGE JUICE
SELTZER

CONDIMENTS

LITE SALAD DRESSING
VINEGAR
PEPPER

GIVE YOUR CHILD THE TITLE OF "THE JUNK FOOD BUSTER"

Tell your child that at the supermarket, he or she is going to turn into "THE JUNK FOOD BUSTER". The child will suddenly realize the adventure, and assume an identity similar to that of a cartoon super hero.

The mission of "THE JUNK FOOD BUSTER" is to select healthy foods for the entire family. Therefore, not allowing any junk food (food which is high in calories, fat, or sugar) to pass the way of "THE JUNK FOOD BUSTER". A child will love the opportunity to help out and search for foods that are on the shopping list.

One particular game which children will enjoy is *I SPY*. One player will give a clue which pertains to a particular food, while the other player must guess which food it is. For example, a parent will say "I SPY with my little eye a food that is in the fruit group which is good for colds and it begins with the letter 'O'". Make sure that while playing *I SPY*, the type of food group is included, and at least one clue which will identify a nutritious aspect.

When food shopping with your child, make certain that either one of you do not go to the supermarket on an empty stomach. Additionally, patience is a must as a child explores each aisle of the supermarket as an *Adventureland* .

Food shopping is also an excellent opportunity for children to sharpen their reading and arithmetic skills. By reading food labels, a child can identify the ingredients, then calculate the number of calories and fat grams.

As adults, we must examine our own attitudes toward food shopping. If we dread food shopping, so will our children. Learn to maintain a healthy outlook for the entire food shopping experience.

SCHOOL TRIP TO THE SUPERMARKET

Plan to bring a school class to the supermarket to study the variety of nutritious food available. This activity may involve a little planning in which the details should be discussed with a supermarket store manager in advance.

Going to the supermarket is a great field trip for second grade level students and older. A trip of this type will enhance the overall knowledge of food and nutrition. Parents can plan individual trips as well.

Preparing for such a field trip is very important. Make sure that the children have a basic understanding of proper nutrition. Prior to the trip, children should receive an overview of the four food groups, foods which are high in fat, sugar, and cholesterol. Additionally, a lesson on how to read and comprehend food labels would create a good foundation to build on.

Divide the class into six groups. Each group will be told to make a food list from each food group. Each list should contain between five to ten items. Detailed below is an example of how the six groups are each given a shopping cart, and how each group is given a specific food category.

GROUP #1   FRUITS
GROUP #2   VEGETABLES
GROUP #3   DAIRY
GROUP #4   MEATS / PROTEIN
GROUP #5   BREADS / CEREALS
GROUP #6   JUNK FOODS (High in fat, sugar, and cholesterol)

The children can search for the foods which pertain to their specific lists. Each group is given twenty-five minutes to look for the various foods that apply to them. When the twenty-five minutes are over, all the groups can meet in a designated area within the supermarket. The teacher, students, and escorts (if available) will review the contents in each shopping cart. With the exception of the junk foods, the most nutritional aspects of each food should be discussed. If a child has chosen a food which is considered high in fat, sugar, or cholesterol, he or she can be told to exchange the item with a similar product which is more acceptable. For example, whole milk should be exchanged for skim milk, and sugar cereal can be exchanged with wheat flakes. In regard to the shopping cart containing the junk foods, all of the unhealthy ingredients can be discussed.

Children love this activity because it allows them to be in control of the shopping cart. Although that aspect may not seem like a lot to an adult, a child may realize a greater sense of maturity afterward.

CHAPTER 13
FIT-KID CHEF

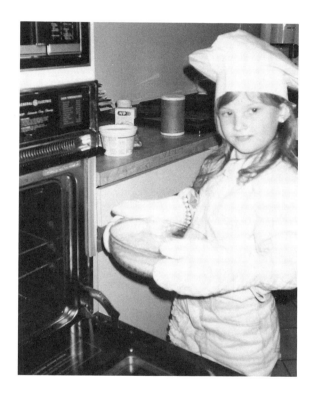

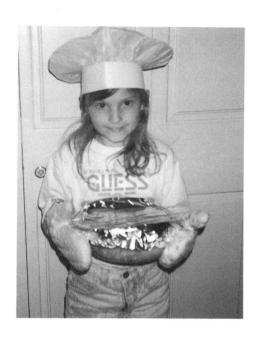

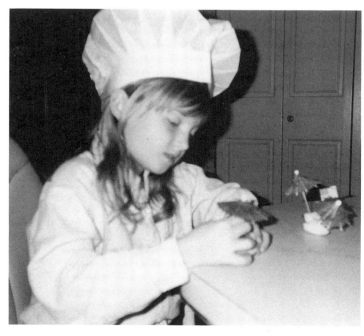

Thirteen

Between the ages of four and eleven, both girls and boys require a minimal amount of encouragement to become involved with cooking. Some parents view cooking as a chore. However, children perceive the various aspects of cooking as exciting. Moreover, children may see mixing, measuring, stirring, and tasting as a form of play.

Allowing the child to be involved with cooking will stimulate maturity, and raise consciousness on the benefits of eating healthy. Let him or her become an integral part of the cooking process at home. Give the child the honor of becoming a "FIT-KID Chef". Imagine the boost to the sense of accomplishment and level of confidence when a child serves dishes he or she has prepared. Children will become more willing to eat meals that are new to their menu if they are actively involved in the preparation. Additionally, they will learn the value of good nutrition. Having the child assist in setting and clearing the table will also help instill confidence and provide another venue for maturity.

As children become more involved with cooking, they will develop other skills such as reading (recipes and labels), basic mathematics (measuring and timing foods), and coordination (pouring, mixing, and cutting). I have also found that supplying a child with a personalized set of measuring utensils will enhance his or her sense of importance.

Perhaps the most important benefit of cooking with a "FIT-KID Chef" is the quality time which can be shared. Allowing the child to be independent as well as part of a team in the kitchen can be an enjoyable learning experience for everyone involved.

Prior to beginning any of the cooking adventures mentioned within this chapter, it must be emphasized that adult supervision is an absolute necessity. In the interest of safety, it is always advisable to assist children with the use of electrical appliances, ovens, stoves, and sharp implements.

This chapter introduces many FIT-KID, "kid-tested" recipes. These meals have been designed to be fun and easy, but moreover, to help the child (and "grown-up" assistant) realize the importance of maintaining a healthy diet.

Although it is important to follow directions, it can also be fun for the child to experiment and become imaginative with these recipes.

Art is as important as science in the real world. There have been great discoveries realized from mistakes. By experimenting, the child will discover there is more than one way to prepare a dish.

BRIGHT BEGINNINGS

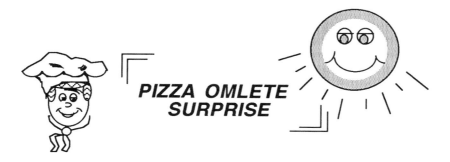

PIZZA OMLETE SURPRISE

1 egg, plus 2 egg whites

1/4 cup skim milk

Dash each salt and pepper

1 slice of mozzarella cheese

1/4 cup tomato sauce

oregano (to desired taste)

mushrooms sliced

Preheat a 10-inch nonstick omelet pan (or skillet sprayed with nonstick cooking spray) at low setting.

In a small mixing bowl combine eggs, milk, salt, and pepper, and beat until whipped; pour in egg mixture and cook until the bottom of the omelet solidifies. Arrange tomato sauce, cheese, mushrooms, and oregano over half of omelet; fold other half over and heat for approximately 1 minute. Carefully slide omelet onto platter or use a spatula to lift out of skillet. Makes 1 serving.

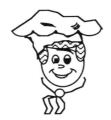

EGG ON A NEST

1 slice of bread (light or regular) whole wheat

1 egg and 1 egg white

1/4 cup of low fat milk

1 slice of light cheese (your choice)

Preheat a nonstick frying pan at low setting. In a small mixing bowl combine egg, egg white, and low fat milk; beat until whipped. Cut hole in center of bread slice. Toast bread until lightly golden.

Pour egg mixture into frying pan and scramble until cooked. Remove from pan and place the scrambled egg into the hole of the toasted bread. Place the cheese slice on top, and put back into the pan. Cover for 1 minute. Makes 1 serving.

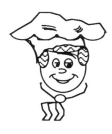

FRENCH TOAST FINGERS

1 egg, and 1 egg white

1/4 cup low fat milk

1 teaspoon vanilla

1 teaspoon ground cinnamon

2 slices of bread

Preheat a nonstick frying pan at low setting. Slice bread into 5 strips. In shallow bowl combine eggs, milk, vanilla, and cinnamon. Dip bread slices into egg mixture, coating all sides; let bread soak in mixture until as much liquid as possible has been absorbed.

Place bread slices into frying pan and cook until bread is browned on underside; turn slices and brown other side. To serve, place syrup in a plastic cup, and let the child dip away. Makes 2 servings.

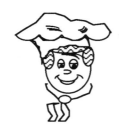

MICKEY PANCAKES

1 cup whole wheat flour

1 cup unbleached flour

11/2 cups buttermilk

1 teaspoon sugar

1 teaspoon baking soda

1 teaspoon baking powder

2 eggs

2 teaspoons light cooking oil

pineapple slices

cherry slices

Preheat a griddle at low setting. In medium bowl beat eggs until fluffy; alternately beat in flour, baking soda, baking powder, buttermilk, sugar, and oil. Pour batter onto griddle and cook until bottom side of pancake is golden. Use a spatula to turn over and cook other side.

Arrange the fruit slices over each pancake to form a face; use 2 halves of a cherry for eyes, and 1 half of a pineapple slice for a smile.

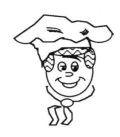

FRESH APPLE CUPCAKES

2/3 cup all purpose flour

1/3 cup whole wheat flour

1/3 cup sugar

1/2 teaspoon baking soda

1/2 teaspoon ground ginger

1/3 cup vegetable oil

1 egg

1 1/2 cup corded chopped apple (peeled)

1 teaspoon vanilla extract

Preheat oven to 350 degrees F. In medium mixing bowl combine flour, sugar, baking soda, and ginger. Then add oil, egg, apple, and vanilla. Stir until mixture forms a sticky dough.

Line a 6 muffin pan with muffin cups. Spoon an equal amount of mixture into each cup. Bake until cupcakes are golden brown, approximately 35 minutes.

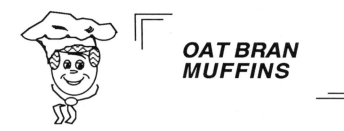

OAT BRAN MUFFINS

2 cups oat bran cereal

1/4 cup brown sugar

2 teaspoons baking powder

1 cup low fat milk

2 egg whites

1/4 cup honey

2 tablespoons vegetable oil

Preheat oven to 425 degrees F. In medium mixing bowl combine oat bran cereal, brown sugar, baking powder. Add milk, egg whites, honey, and oil. Stir until mixture forms a sticky dough.

Spray twelve 2 1/2-inch-diameter muffin pan cups with nonstick cooking spray; Spoon an equal amount of mixture into each cup. Bake until muffins are golden brown, 18 to 20 minutes.

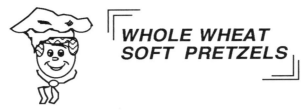

WHOLE WHEAT SOFT PRETZELS

1 package active dry yeast

1 1/2 cups warm water

2 3/4 cups all-purpose

3 teaspoons sugar

1/2 teaspoon salt

1 to 1 1/2 cups whole wheat flour

1 egg

1 tablespoon cold water

2 tablespoons coarse salt

Dissolve yeast in warm water. Add all-purpose flour, sugar, and salt. Blend with electric mixer at medium speed. Add whole wheat flour (to make dough easier to manipulate. Place dough onto floured surface and knead until smooth.

Grease sides of a medium size bowl. Place dough into bowl and cover. Allow dough to stand in warm area until it rises to approximately twice the original size (about 1 hour).

Preheat oven to 475 degrees F. Divide dough into two halves. Then cut each half into 6 equal pieces. Roll each piece between palms of hands into 15-inch-long strips (resembling rope).

Place strips of dough on lightly greased cookie sheet. Bring left end of each strip over the middle to form loop. Bring right end of each strip over the first loop to form pretzel shape.

Mix egg with cold water. Brush pretzels with mixture and sprinkle with coarse salt. Bake 15 to 20 minutes. Serves 12.

FAVORITE FIT-KID LUNCHES

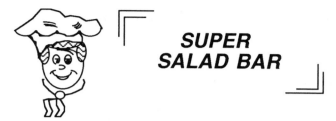

SUPER SALAD BAR

Kids love to create their own combinations, so why not make a salad bar at home? The FIT-KID Chef will enjoy dicing and slicing;

lettuce

celery

mushrooms

zucchini

raisins

tomatoes

peas

croutons

Allow the child to be creative. Various dressings and garnishes may be used as well as different types of colorful platters.

GRILLED CHEESE

Coat frying pan with nonstick butter-flavored cooking spray. Apply a slight amount of the cooking spray to one side of a slice of bread. Place the sprayed side down into the pan. Set at medium heat. Place 1-2 slices of low fat cheese onto bread, and top with another bread slice. Apply a small amount of cooking spray onto the top of the bread. Cook until the underside has been browned. Flip sandwich over and cook other side. You're done!

TUNA SALAD

1 can tuna (solid white, packed in water)

1 celery stick

1 green onion

1/4 cup of low fat mayonnaise

dash salt and pepper

1 teaspoon vinegar

Spread tuna into medium sized bowl. Slice onion and celery, and blend into tuna. Add mayonnaise, salt, pepper, and vinegar. Place on bread (or pita). Cookie cutters may be used to shape the bread into fun figures prior to spreading the tuna salad.

SLOPPY JOANANNES

1 pound ground turkey meat

3/4 cup chopped onion

1 cup ready-made spaghetti sauce

1 teaspoon worchestershire sauce

salt and pepper (to desired taste)

frankfurter or hamburger buns

Preheat skillet at medium temperature. Saute' chopped onion and turkey in skillet until thoroughly cooked. Add remaining ingredients and simmer 15 minutes. Serve on a frankfurter roll or hamburger bun.

PITA POCKET CHEF SALAD SANDWICH BUFFET

2 pita pockets

lettuce

tomato

cheese (your choice)

turkey slices

**1 tablespoon low fat mayonnaise
(or favorite dressing)**

Shred lettuce and slice tomatoes. Slice cheese and turkey into strips. Stuff pita pockets with lettuce, turkey, and cheese, and add dressing. Serve hot or cold. To heat, place pita pocket in microwave for 10 seconds, until cheese is melted.

DELICIOUS DINNERS

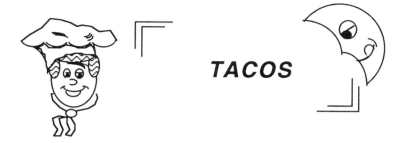

TACOS

taco shells (ready made)

ground turkey

lettuce

tomatoes

4 ounces grated cheddar cheese

plain yogurt

ready made seasonings

Blend seasoning into ground turkey. Preheat skillet at medium temperature.
Saute' turkey in skillet until thoroughly cooked. Place turkey in a serving bowl.
Place shredded lettuce, sliced tomatoes, grated cheese, and yogurt in serving
bowls. Let everyone prepare their own taco (that's half of the fun)!

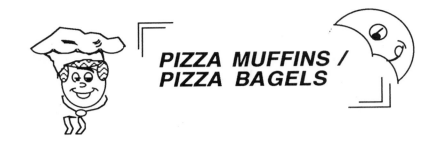

PIZZA MUFFINS / PIZZA BAGELS

2 English muffins or bagels

1/2 cup ready made pizza sauce*

grated mozzarella cheese

oregano

Preheat oven at 400 degrees F. Slice English muffins or bagels down the middle. Toast the muffins in the oven for approximately 20 seconds (bagels will not need to be pre-toasted).

After removing the muffins from the oven, spread pizza sauce on top of each 1/2 of muffin or bagel. Sprinkle cheese on each half and add oregano. Bake until cheese melts.

* pizza sauce may be substituted with plain spaghetti sauce.

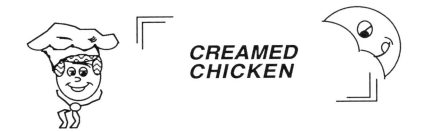

CREAMED CHICKEN

1 pound boneless chicken breasts

1 can of cream of mushroom soup

1/2 cup of milk

Slice chicken breasts into cubes and boil in water for 15 minutes. Heat soup and stir in milk. Place cooked chicken in soup and simmer for 10 minutes. Serve over cooked rice or egg noodles. Serves 3.

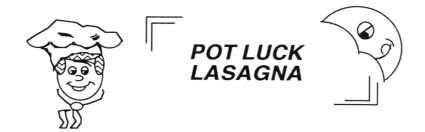

POT LUCK LASAGNA

8 ounces macaroni or colored spiral pasta

2 teaspoons oregano

1 jar tomato sauce

2 cups low fat ricotta cheese

1/2 cup parmesan cheese

8 ounces mozzarella cheese

Cook pasta in boiling water until tender, then drain. In a large mixing bowl, blend in pasta, oregano, tomato sauce, ricotta cheese, and parmesan cheese. Preheat oven to 375 degrees F.

Place mixed ingredients into a baking dish and spread mozzarella cheese over the top. Bake for 15 minutes.

Serves 4.

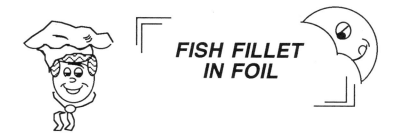

FISH FILLET IN FOIL

4 four-to-six ounce fish fillets

2 medium potatoes (peeled, thinly sliced)

4 teaspoons margarine

1 carrot (sliced thin)

Preheat oven to 375 degrees F.

Cut 4 8-inch-by-12-inch pieces of aluminum foil. Place one piece of foil on a clean surface with shiny side down (when folded inward, shiny side will be on exterior).

Place approximately one-fourth of the potato slices in the center of the foil. Add 1/2 teaspoon of margarine. Place a fish fillet on top.

Layer approximately one-fourth of the carrot slices on top of the fish fillet. Add another 1/2 teaspoon of margarine on top of the carrots.

Fold foil over ingredients loosely. Prepare all 4 identically.

Place the foil envelopes onto a cookie sheet and bake for 20 minutes.

141

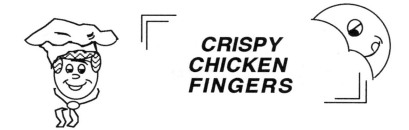

CRISPY CHICKEN FINGERS

4 boneless chicken breasts

1 cup corn flake crumbs

2 egg whites

1/8 cup skim milk

1 packet chicken powder

Preheat oven to 375 degrees F.

Mix milk and egg whites together. Combine corn flake crumbs and chicken powder; pour mixture onto sheet of wax paper or paper plate.

Slice chicken into long strips and dip into egg mixture. Roll chicken into crumb mixture. Place chicken strips onto a nonstick cookie sheet.

Bake for 30 minutes. May be served with vegetable, rice, or baked potato.

Serves 4.

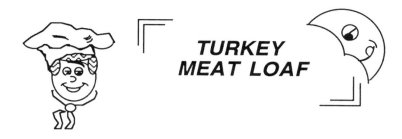

TURKEY MEAT LOAF

1 pound ground turkey

3/4 cup tomato sauce

3/4 cup uncooked oatmeal (or unprocessed bran)

2 egg whites

1/2 diced onion

dash salt & pepper

1/4 teaspoon oregano

Preheat oven to 350 degrees F.

In medium bowl combine all ingredients; shape into a loaf. Transfer to 9-inch-by-5-inch loaf pan, and bake for 1 hour.

Serves 4 to 6.

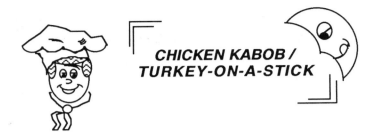

**CHICKEN KABOB /
TURKEY-ON-A-STICK**

1/2 pound boneless chicken breasts

OR

1/2 pound turkey dogs

2 carrots

Slice chicken breasts into cubes and boil in water for 15 minutes / boil turkey dogs in water until tender. Boil carrots in water until tender.

Slice cooked chicken / turkey dogs, and carrots.   Place alternately on kabob sticks. May be served accompanied with paper cups filled with tomato catsup or mustard for dipping.

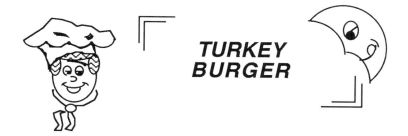

TURKEY BURGER

1 pound ground turkey

2 egg whites

1 chicken bullion packet

1/4 cup unprocessed bran

Combine all ingredients and form 4 patties. Cook in frying pan until brown.

Melt low fat cheese on top of the patties if desired. May be served on light

hamburger buns. Serves 4.

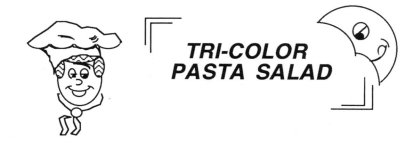

TRI-COLOR PASTA SALAD

8 ounces cooked tricolored pasta, chilled

celery (sliced thin)

tomatoes (sliced and diced)

dash salt and pepper

1 1/2 teaspoons vinegar

3 tablespoons plain yogurt

2 tablespoons lite thousand island, or French dressing

In bowl combine all ingredients and toss until well mixed; cover and refrigerate for 1 hour. Toss again before serving. Makes 4 servings.

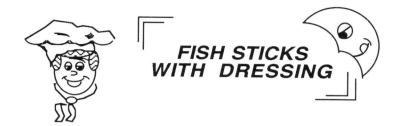

FISH STICKS WITH DRESSING

1 pound flounder

4 cups crushed corn flakes

3 egg whites

1/4 cup milk

dash salt and pepper

1 packet chicken powder

freshly squeezed lemon juice

ketchup or lite dressing

Preheat oven to 350 degrees F. Rinse fish in cold water, slice into strips, and set aside.

In a bowl combine crushed corn flakes and chicken powder; mix well. In a separate bowl combine egg whites, milk, salt, and pepper. Pour lemon juice over fish strips, and dip fish in egg mixture; transfer to nonstick baking sheet. Bake 15 minutes.

Fill paper cups with ketchup or lite dressing for dipping. Serve with rice.

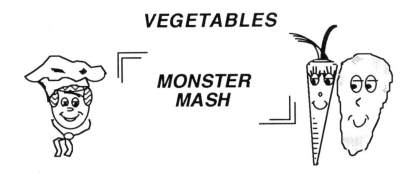

VEGETABLES

MONSTER MASH

one pound raw potatoes

2 teaspoons butter

Wash potatoes; peel and cut into chunks. Add potatoes to 1 1/2 cups cold water,
and cook thoroughly; drain water. Mash potatoes in separate bowl using
electric mixer. Add salt, pepper, and butter to desired taste.

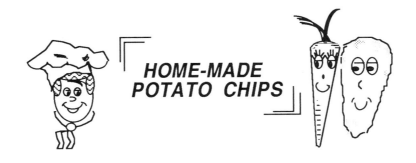

HOME-MADE POTATO CHIPS

1 pound potatoes

2 tablespoons oil

Preheat oven to 400 degrees F. Slice potatoes to paper thin size; spread slices out in single layers on lightly oiled baking sheet.

Bake 15 to 20 minutes until potatoes are golden brown. Add salt and pepper to desired taste.

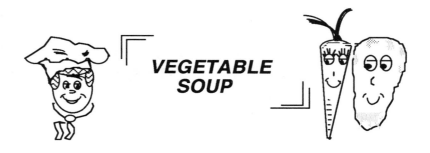

VEGETABLE SOUP

4 packets chicken or beef broth

1/2 cup coarsely chopped onion

1/2 cup each sliced carrots and potatoes

1/2 cup each cut green beans, peas, and turnips

1/2 cup rice

Add all ingredients to large pot of water. Cook over medium heat, stirring occasionally; bring to a boil. Reduce heat, cover, and let simmer for 30 - 40 minutes, stirring occasionally. The types of vegetables are optional and may be substituted.

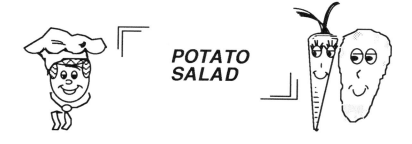

POTATO SALAD

2 large red potatoes

2 green onions chopped

2 celery stalks chopped

1/8 teaspoon salt

1/8 teaspoon pepper

3 tablespoons plain yogurt

1 tablespoon lite thousand island dressing, or 3 tablespoons lite mayonnaise

Wash potatoes;cut into chunks (peeling is optional). Add potatoes to 1 1/2 cups cold water, and cook thoroughly (approximately 20 minutes); drain water. Chill the cooked potatoes approximately 1 hour. Blend the onions, celery, yogurt, dressing / mayonnaise, salt, and pepper into the chilled potatoes. Keep chilled until served.

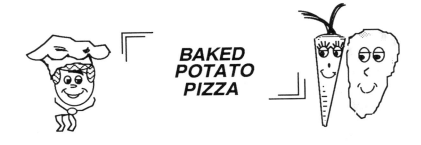

BAKED POTATO PIZZA

4 large potatoes

3/4 cup grated mozzarella cheese

1/2 cup parmesan cheese

1/2 cup low fat / skim milk

3/4 cup tomato sauce

Preheat oven to 375 degrees F. Puncture each potato with several fork holes before baking. Bake potatoes in oven approximately 45 minutes, until cooked. (For microwave cooking, puncture potatoes and cook on high setting for 20 - 30 minutes, rotating each potato after 10 - 15 minutes of cooking.

Cut one end off each potato to create an opening. Scoop out the inside of each potato. In a bowl combine potatoes, parmesan and mozzarella cheese, and milk; mix well. Pour small amount of tomato sauce into empty shells, and add potato mixture to fill each one. Sprinkle 1 tablespoon of mozzarella on top of each potato. Heat in oven at low setting until cheese melts. Heat remaining sauce; pour over potatoes or serve as side dish.

152

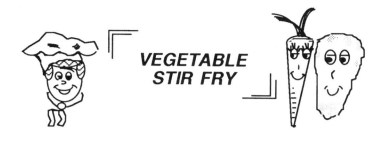

VEGETABLE STIR FRY

1/2 cup orange juice

1/4 cup water

1 tablespoon low sodium soy sauce

2 tablespoons white vinegar

1 tablespoon cornstarch

1 tablespoon vegetable oil

1 medium carrot sliced thin

1 green pepper / 1 red pepper

shredded cabbage

fresh or frozen snow peas

1 can mandarin oranges

1/2 cup canned sliced water chestnuts

8 ears barley corn

4 scallions trimmed and thinly sliced

cooked rice

In a bowl combine orange juice, water, soy sauce vinegar, and cornstarch; mix well. Heat vegetable oil in frying pan and add vegetables alternately. Add cornstarch mixture to vegetables; stir until mixture thickens to a sauce. Serve over cooked rice. Serves 4.

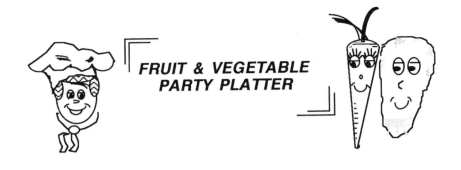

FRUIT & VEGETABLE PARTY PLATTER

celery (cut pieces to 2 inch length)

apples (cut into wedges)

cucumbers (cut round slices)

lettuce leaves

Combine fruits and vegetables (using any desired variations) cut into various shapes and sizes. Garnish with lettuce leaves and serve on a party platter.

FOR SPREADS

lite cream cheese

peanut butter

cheese spread (of choice)

FOR TOPPINGS

raisins

sunflower seeds

granola

To enhance your vegetable and fruit platter, try filling an icing bag with cheese spread, and creating your own unique and attractive designs. Children will really enjoy this too!

SLICED VEGETABLE PLATTER WITH DIP

sliced carrot sticks

sliced cucumber

raw broccoli stalks

raw cauliflower stalks

1 cup plain yogurt

1 packet onion bullion powder

In a small bowl combine yogurt and onion powder, to form dip. Arrange sliced vegetables creatively on a platter and serve.

BAKED POTATO

1 large potato

1/2 cup plain yogurt / cottage cheese / low calorie dressing

Preheat oven to 375 degrees F. Puncture potato with several fork holes before baking. Bake potato in oven approximately 25 minutes, until cooked. (For microwave cooking, puncture potatoes and cook on high setting for 8 - 10 minutes, rotating after 5 minutes of cooking.

Slice potato open and fill with favorite topping (avoid using butter).

DESSERTS

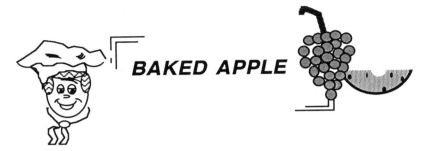

BAKED APPLE

1 **large baking apple**
1 **tablespoon raisins**
1/2 **cup seltzer**
1 1/2 **teaspoons sugar**

Core apple and place in bowl. Pour seltzer into hole of apple. Sprinkle cinnamon and sugar over apple. Pour raisins into hole of apple. Preheat oven to 375 degrees F. Bake apple in oven approximately 20 minutes, until cooked. (For microwave cooking, cook on high setting for 5 - 7 minutes, rotating after 3 minutes of cooking. Top with a spoonful of plain yogurt. Serves 1.

APPLE PITA PIE

8 **apples**
3 **pitas**
3/4 **cup water**
1 **teaspoon sugar**
cinnamon

Peel and slice apples. Cook apples in water with sugar added until tender (but not soggy). Drain, then cool. Add cinnamon to apples and spoon into pitas. Serves 3.

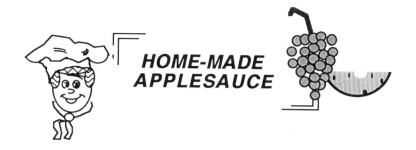

HOME-MADE APPLESAUCE

5 baking apples

1/2 cup water

1 teaspoon cinnamon

3 tablespoons sugar

Peel and core apples. Place apples into saucepan and add water and cinnamon. Cook until apples are tender enough to mash easily. Mash apples using a potato masher; add sugar. Serve warm or cold. Serves 4.

CHEERIOS NECKLACE

1 cup Cheerios cereal

1 spool of string (bakery type)

Thread Cheerios onto string forming a necklace. Tie ends of string together. A fun and nutritious activity.

157

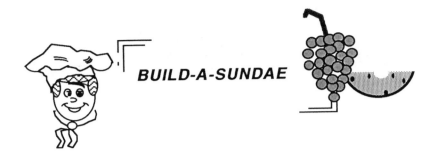

BUILD-A-SUNDAE

1 cup yogurt (vanilla or fruit)

1 pound chopped fruits (desired mix such as: apples, melons, raisins, etc.)

1/8 cup chopped nuts

2 bananas

Spoon yogurt, fruit, and nuts into individual plastic glasses. Slice bananas down the middle. Help yourself to a buffet-style sundae treat!

PEANUT BUTTER BALLS

1/2 cup peanut butter (creamy style)

1/4 cup honey

1/2 teaspoon vanilla

2-to-3 cups Rice Krispies cereal

Combine peanut butter, honey, and vanilla. Stir in cereal. Moisten hands and form mixture into balls. Place onto waxed paper and chill.

158

PARTY RECIPES

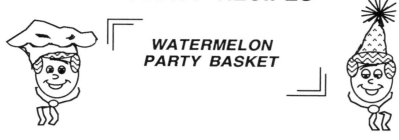

WATERMELON PARTY BASKET

Slice whole watermelon into a basket shape. Remove inside of watermelon with a scoop to form melon balls. Place the melon balls back into the "basket". Add a variety of whole fruit (cherries, grapes, etc.) and sliced fruit (banana, cantaloupe, etc.).

HAWAIIAN FRUIT BUSH

1 pineapple (whole)

1 pound grapes (seedless)

1 pound cheese (unsliced; your choice)

sweet pickles (sliced)

Slice cheese into cubes. Place cheese cubes onto toothpicks, followed by grapes and sweet pickles creating toothpick kabob. Place filled toothpicks into pineapple. This makes a fun party centerpiece. If a pineapple is unavailable, a grapefruit may be substituted.

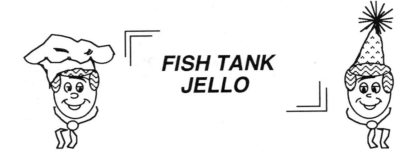

FISH TANK JELLO

Make gelatin dessert according to package directions. Blueberry flavor can be used to simulate the ocean. Once refrigerated, the gelatin will begin to jell. Add gummy fish to each serving cup or bowl. The fish will become suspended in the center of the dessert creating an edible fish tank.

FRUIT YOGURT FUN-FIT POPS

6 ounces orange juice

6 ounces water

1 cup non-fat plain yogurt

1 teaspoon vanilla

Combine all ingredients into a blender. Blend at low setting for approximately 2 minutes. Pour mixture into paper cups. Place a plastic spoon into the cups and freeze for several hours.

To vary this dessert, just use your favorite juices without the addition of other ingredients.

160

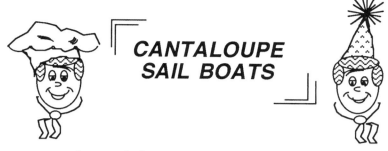

CANTALOUPE SAIL BOATS

1 cantaloupe

1/2 pound grapes (seedless)

1/2 pound cherries

1 can pineapple slices

1 pound cheese (unsliced; your choice)

Cut cantaloupe first in half; then cut each half into three slices. Slice cheese into cubes. Place cheese cubes onto toothpicks, followed by grapes, cherries, pineapple cubes, or a variation of other pieces of fruit creating toothpick kabob. Place filled toothpicks into the center of the cantaloupe slices.

FRUIT DIPS

Using either kabob sticks or swizzle sticks (approximately 5-inches in length), place cheese cubes onto sticks; followed by grapes, cherries, pineapple cubes, or a variation of other pieces of fruit creating fruit kabob. Dip the fruit kabob into a 1/2 cup of your favorite yogurt or you can create a MAPLE YOGURT DIPPING SAUCE;

2 tablespoons low fat plain yogurt

3 ounces light cream cheese

1 tablespoon maple syrup

Blend ingredients and place into a bowl for dipping.

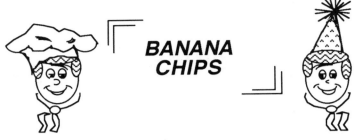

BANANA CHIPS

4 bananas

1/4 cup lemon juice

Preheat oven at 175 degrees F. Slice bananas and dip into lemon juice. Place on a nonstick cookie sheet in a single layer. Bake for approximately 2-to-3 hours until golden brown. Store in an airtight container.

CEREAL NIBBLES

5 cups mixed dry cereal

2 cups broken pretzels

1/3 cup corn oil margarine

4 teaspoons worchestershire sauce

1 teaspoon celery flakes

1/2 teaspoon onion powder

1/2 teaspoon garlic powder

1 cup mixed nuts

Preheat oven at 275 degrees F. Combine dry cereal and pretzels. Melt margarine in saucepan and combine with worchestershire sauce and seasonings. Place in a shallow roasting pan and bake for approximately 1 hour.

BEVERAGES

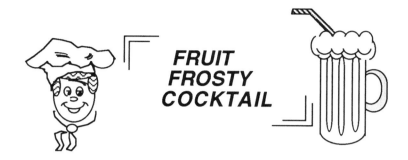

FRUIT FROSTY COCKTAIL

1/2 cup ice cubes

1 cup unsweetened pineapple juice

1/2 cup low-fat yogurt (plain or fruit)

1/2 cup fruit (your choice)

Place all ingredients into a blender. Cover and blend until a smooth texture is achieved. Pour mixture into a fancy glass with a slice of pineapple or miniature umbrella.

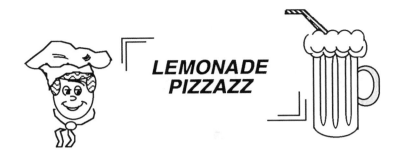

LEMONADE PIZZAZZ

1/4 cup freshly squeezed lemon juice

1 tablespoon sugar

3/4 cup seltzer

ice cubes

lemon slice

Combine lemon juice and sugar. Add water and ice cubes; mix. Pour mixture into a fancy glass with a slice of lemon. Makes 1 serving.

ORANGE PIZZAZZ

12 ounces orange juice

12 ounces seltzer

Mix and serve. Makes 3 servings.

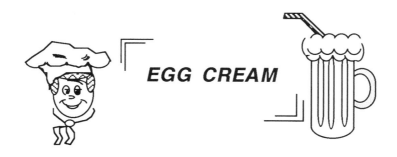

EGG CREAM

1 cup seltzer

3/4 cup skim milk

1/2 teaspoon vanilla extract

2-to-3 teaspoons sugar

2 ice cubes

Combine ingredients into blender. Mix until smooth. Makes 1 serving.

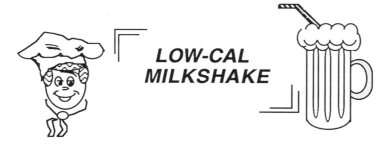

LOW-CAL MILKSHAKE

1 cup low fat milk

1 teaspoon vanilla extract

2-to-3 teaspoons sugar

2-to-3 ice cubes

Combine ingredients into blender. Mix until smooth. Makes 1 serving.

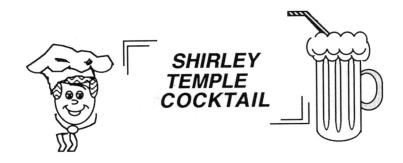

SHIRLEY TEMPLE COCKTAIL

1 cup seltzer

1/4 cup cranberry juice

Mix ingredients. Serve in a fancy glass. Add cherry / miniature umbrella.

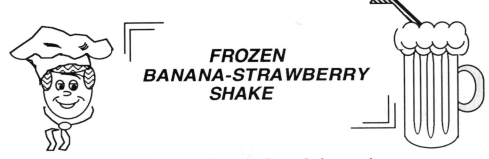

FROZEN BANANA-STRAWBERRY SHAKE

1 banana (peeled and frozen)

6 strawberries

1/4 cup low fat vanilla yogurt

1 tablespoon cranberry juice

Blend all ingredients. Pour into a fancy glass. Garnish with a strawberry.

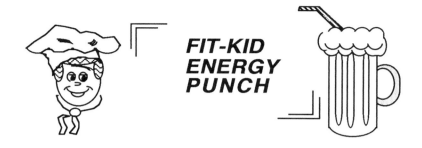

FIT-KID ENERGY PUNCH

1/4 gallon orange juice

2 cups pineapple juice

1 cup pineapple chunks

1/2 cup cherries

2 oranges (sliced)

1 tray ice cubes

Combine all ingredients into a punch bowl or pitcher.

"JUICE-IT"

A wise investment to be considered is a juicer. Kids love to create their own juice. Allowing children to be involved in the production process is an excellent way to replenish the fluids necessary after a workout. Several fresh juice ideas that can be delicious and nutritious are;

carrot juice

tomato juice

orange juice

apple juice

pineapple juice

CHAPTER 14
FOOD FIT FOR A KID

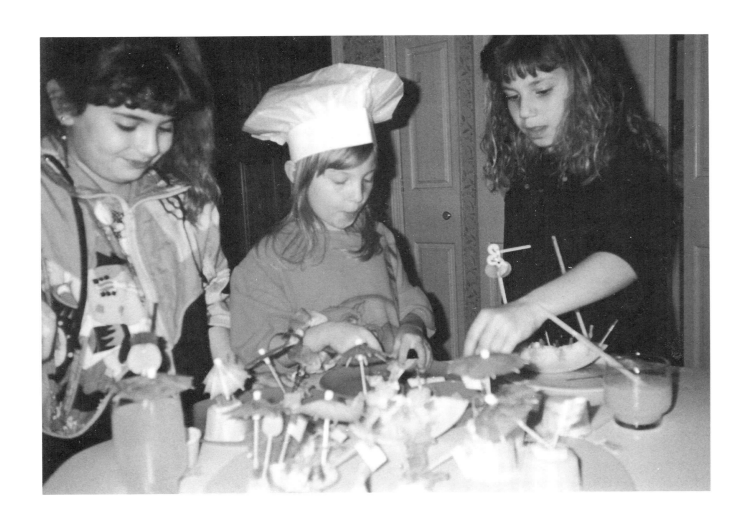

Fourteen

"Sell the sizzle, not the steak" is an approach often used by marketing experts in the media. Advertisers specializing in children's television commercials sell adventure and fun. Children become mesmerized by dancing bears selling cereal or the adventure of finding the hidden cookie in Cookieland. These are examples of exciting concepts to achieve the acceptance of children. When the child becomes receptive to the message of the advertiser, he or she will try to convince the parent to purchase the product. The same techniques that entice children to eat junk food can be used equally well to have them become involved in eating healthy food.

A scene all too common in supermarkets is a child *dragging* the parent down the cereal aisle toward the most colorful boxes. The cereal with the best jingle or free prize also receives the most attention. Parents usually appease the demands of the child. Getting a child to eat can be difficult. Parents are relieved when the child becomes attracted to a particular food. Once home, the child cannot wait to tear open the box to search for the *buried treasure* .

I have worked with children for seven years as well as having a child of my own. It has been a fascinating experience studying children and their eating habits.

Most fast food restaurants offer variations of a meal designed specifically for children. The meal is usually referred to with an attractive name (such as a *fun meal*), as well using colorful boxes, animated characters, and sometimes an added toy.

One study I have conducted took place at a fast food restaurant. I surveyed the participating children individually to see if they would prefer a hamburger, French fries, and a soft drink or a *fun meal* as an alternative. Every child requested a *fun meal*.

When I inquired why they wanted the *fun meal*, I received answers like "because it tastes better", "it has a prize", and "it comes in a box". It is ironic how children believe the exact same meal tastes better if it presented more attractively and offers a prize.

Another example of how packaging and presentation can be responsible for one-hundred percent difference in a child's attitude toward food is the *taste test*. This can be an interesting activity to try with a child or a group of children (a group of children would provide credence of peer pressure).

I had organized a taste test with a group of children that participate in my FIT-KID programs. I had placed a popular brand cereal in a glass bowl next to the exact same brand still in the colorful cardboard box. Each child took a sample from both the bowl, and then the box. When questioned, the children agreed that the boxed cereal tasted better. This is a classic example of how the visual stimulus influences of the taste buds.

The same idea may be applied to beverages. I tested a group of children between the ages of five and ten years of age. Several plain glasses were filled with orange juice. While an equal number of glasses with lids and straws (the type frequently used at fast food restaurants) were also filled with the same type of orange juice. I asked the children to first taste the juice in the regular glasses, and then try the juice in the glasses with the lids and straws. After surveying the comments of the children, it was overwhelmingly agreed that the orange juice with the lids and straws tasted better.

I had prepared a buffet lunch for a group of children which consisted of similar types of food, but prepared differently. The following two sets of food were presented, and are categorized simply as "creative" and "plain";

<table>
<tr><td>CREATIVE</td><td>PLAIN</td></tr>
<tr><td>• Fresh fruit in a watermelon basket.</td><td>• Sliced fruit in a plate.</td></tr>
<tr><td>• Salad with assorted dressings in bottles on the side.</td><td>• Previously dressed salad.</td></tr>
<tr><td>• Assorted sandwiches shaped with cookie cutters.</td><td>• Sandwiches cut diagonally.</td></tr>
<tr><td>• Fruit juice in a punch bowl with slices of pineapple and cherries accompanied with a fancy ladle and plastic wine glasses.</td><td>• Cups of soda.</td></tr>
<tr><td>• Granola snacks placed in Dixie cups.</td><td>• One bowl of potato chips.</td></tr>
</table>

The children were left alone and allowed to serve themselves. The children gravitated toward the more creative snacks. The food that was more appealing to the eye was almost completely finished compared to the plain food. The self-serve factor also played a large part in attracting the attention of the children. It is likely that using the ladle instilled a level of confidence and maturity.

171

In order to promote healthy eating habits to children, food should be appetizing, tasty, and nutritious. Developing tasty meals and snacks does not necessarily mean the addition of herbs and spices. Children will be interested in meals that are well presented. Moreover, an amusing table setting can spark the appetite of a child.

As adults, we have realized the importance of attractive table settings for dining. An example of this fact is demonstrated when adults enjoy going out to dinner to an elegant restaurant. If adults are treated to exquisite motivation factors such as center pieces and fancy food arrangements, why shouldn't children have the same privilege?

In the previous chapter, FIT-KID CHEF, many healthy (and fun to make) recipes were presented for both the adult and child. This chapter will demonstrate how to add excitement into mealtime. By simply adding several creative ideas involving presentation, the average meal or snack can receive a dramatic lift.

Listed on the following page are many items which can bring instant excitement to the dinner table for children. Many items can be easily found at a supermarket, or a store specializing in party materials.

- [ ] TOOTHPICKS WITH FLAGS
- [ ] TOOTHPICKS WITH COLOR OR DESIGNS
- [ ] UMBRELLA TOOTHPICKS
- [ ] SECTIONED PAPER / PLASTIC PLATES (DINNER SIZE)
- [ ] SECTIONED BUFFET PLATES
- [ ] COLORFUL PAPER LUNCH BAGS
- [ ] PLASTIC SPOONS, FORKS, KNIVES
- [ ] PLASTIC WINE GLASSES
- [ ] PLASTIC / PAPER CUPS
- [ ] CRAZY STRAWS
- [ ] STRAW
- [ ] ZIP-LOCK BAGGIES
- [ ] COLORFUL PLASTIC BOWLS AND PLATES
- [ ] COLORFUL PLACE MATS
- [ ] PLASTIC PITCHER
- [ ] COLORFUL PLASTIC FOOD CONTAINERS WITH LIDS
- [ ] PLASTIC WATER WORKOUT BOTTLES
- [ ] STAR STICKERS (VARIOUS DESIGNS)

There are many ways to create an exciting ambiance that would encourage a child to eat healthy. All of the techniques mentioned throughout this chapter have been "kid-tested".

A particularly interesting observation I have made involves kids of all ages and their fascination with frozen dinners. I discovered the attraction was not the food contained in the dinner. Instead, the novelty was eating from a plate with sections. The sectioned plate creates an additional element of intrigue and excitement, by offering more choices for the child. Some of the frozen dinners available for children offer an additional incentive such as a prize. The same methods of serving an exciting meal to a child may be achieved at home. A variety of healthy recipes can be served in sectioned plates (colors and designs are also helpful). Bright-colored bowls can be used to serve cereal and soups. As for a prize, a little subtlety goes a long way. "Stickers" depicting animated characters are inexpensive and are always a big hit!

The following serving suggestions for beverages have proven quite successful. Serving water, milk, and juice in the unique ways mentioned below will make it easy for children to drink healthy, and make carbonated soft drinks a thing of the past.

- Dixie cups / plastic cups with animated characters used to serve beverages (or snacks in a buffet style).
- *Crazy Straws* or regular straws.
- Plastic wine glasses (provides a sense of maturity).
- Plastic workout water bottles (one of the most popular methods of getting a child to drink, as well as being extremely accessible).
- A slice of fruit floating on top of a serving of a fruit juice of your choice.
- Miniature umbrella placed into a glass of juice

There are many ways to prepare meals for children (and the rest of the family too) which promote healthy and enjoyable eating habits. It is important (and fun) to break away from the traditional routines of how meals are served in general, and especially to a child. For example, prepare the portions in advance for the child on a plate. By predetermining the amount of food, the child will not over-eat. Additionally, the child will not acquire the habit of wasting food.

The following methods of presenting meals are often taken for granted. With just a little creativity and effort, every meal can be turned into a fun-filled (and healthy) event:

- Family Buffet: A variety of healthy foods may be placed in attractive bright-colored platters on one table or counter top. The children pass along the buffet line serving themselves. The children learn the valuable lesson of making their own nutritional choices.

- Picnics: Just the name alone sounds fun! Who said a picnic is strictly for the sunny outdoors? It can be as enjoyable to plan an indoor picnic. Several nutritious meals can be easily prepared and stored into colorful plastic containers. The filled containers can then be placed into a basket. Spreading a blanket onto the floor of the living room or den can become a group event while preparing an indoor picnic. A picnic can be produced anywhere children find it exciting. It may even be right outside your back door. Allowing the child share in the decision of a picnic location is always a good idea. This will promote self confidence in children as well as maturity. Children enjoy being a part of the decision making process.

Snacking is an inevitable part of a diet for children. The following list is a useful guide of healthy snacks for kids. It is important to make sure that all snacks are prepared and packaged in creative ways.

- Rice cakes alone or used in a peanut butter and jelly configuration.
- Bread sticks.
- Unsweetened cereal.
- Muffins (low cholesterol)
- Carrot sticks (make sure the carrots have bright, fresh appearance and are sliced creatively into sticks).
- Celery boats (add cream cheese and toothpick flags).
- Zucchini sticks.
- Broccoli trees.
- Apple boats (add toothpick flags)
- Orange and pear boats.
- Pineapple slices, or cubes.
- Grapes and cherries (bunches are recommended since children love to pick).
- Low fat cheeses in cubes (kabob sticks can be a fun variation).

It is always a good idea to make fruit and vegetable snacks accessible. Many times, the term *"out of sight, out of mind"* can be applied to fruits and vegetables that are stored into the bins of the refrigerator. In fact, there is no point in purchasing them unless a little extra effort is applied into cleaning, preparing, and packaging the healthy snacks that can be easily accessed by a child. Colorful plastic containers used to store fruit and vegetables accompanied with yogurt dip will encourage children to indulge without hesitation.

176

- School Lunches: Meals at fast food restaurants which are especially designed for children (*fun meals*) are visually stimulating. In addition, the element of surprise is sometimes added when a toy prize, game, or puzzle is included.

When a lunch is prepared for a child to bring to school, the same principles may be applied. Colorful lunch bags may be purchased, or the child can select a lunch box with a favorite television or cartoon character.

Upon preparation of the meal itself, remember to add a little spark. This can be accomplished by simply changing the way a sandwich is cut. Instead of cutting the sandwich in the conventional manner, a large cookie cutter can be used to create shapes. Variety is also the key as several *ziplock baggies* may store several assorted healthy snacks.

Small prizes can be included to instill confidence and reinforcement. Stickers with stars, designs, or characters, can be an inexpensive yet effective way to say "I'm proud of you!". Hiding the prize somewhere within the lunch bag or box can be an added factor.

Beverages in the school lunch are very important. Recently, there have been many juice companies all using the same concept. Various juices are packaged in small, colorful, single-serving boxes equipped with straws. These containers are very appealing to children.

Once the school lunch has been prepared, tell the child that you have made him or her a special surprise lunch. You may even want to create a little extra *hype* by telling the child of the hidden prize inside the lunch. The anticipation of the child to have the lunch will rise considerably.

• Table setting: The way the table is set for meals in general will help to create a pleasant eating experience for the child. By pretending the kitchen table or dining room table is a restaurant table, dining can become a celebration. Children should be involved in the setting of the table. Besides being an enjoyable experience, the child will learn table setting etiquette and begin to feel more confident and mature.

During breakfast, colorful place mats, flowers in a vase, and folded napkins create a cheerful beginning to the day. A written menu can easily be prepared to enhance the breakfast experience. A typical menu can include a selection of toast, cereal, and eggs. with a choice of beverage (milk and juices are recommended). Breakfast will never be the same when a child learns to order from a menu.

To enhance the table setting for dinner, candles and folded cloth napkins can provide the child with a sense of elegant dining.

The ideas offered in this section are *kid-tested* , and can be used any day of the week.

A buffet prepared for children can be extremely enjoyable. Additionally, offering a variety of healthy choices to children will allow for self-expression and creativity. The various buffet approaches may be used for main meals, parties, or snack time. You can create your own buffet-style restaurant by using Dixie cups and sectioned plates.

- Breakfast buffet: A variation of cereals in separate bowls or Dixie cups can be prepared for a *mix and match* breakfast experience. As a side addition, a selection of sliced fruit can accompany the breakfast buffet. Bananas, strawberries, and raisins are just a few suggestions.
- Fruit and Cheese Buffet: This buffet basically consists of a variety of fruit and low-fat cheeses sliced into cubes. Colorful toothpicks (covered with decorative cellophane if available) can be placed into the cubes for fun and convenient handling.
- Vegetable Buffet: Colorful and creative vegetable arrangements offered with a variety of low-fat dressings and plain yogurt for *fun-dipping* !

Children love to use their hands place food onto a kabob stick. The child can become as creative as he or she wants to be:
- Stick To It: Turkey dog sliced into small, round pieces placed onto kabob sticks. Side cups of mustard and catsup are used for dipping.
- Sliced Fruit On A Stick: Colorful, arrangements of a variety of sliced fruit placed on a kabob stick.
- Vegetables On A Stick: Several types of vegetables may be sliced, then heated in a microwave oven for approximately five minutes. Allow the vegetables to cool. Place the slices on a kabob stick, season to taste (watch that sodium!).
- Toast-on-a-Stick: Make toast the conventional way. Then cut the toast into various shapes using a small sized cookie cutter. Place the toasted shapes onto a kabob stick and alternate between cheese (low-fat) and the toast.

A very important fact to remember is that one of the biggest mistakes a parent can make is to bribe a child to eat everything on the plate. Activity of this type may provide short-term solutions whereas the child in fact *cleaned the plate*. However, over time, the child will come to dislike (and eventually avoid altogether) certain foods they were forced to eat.

A child should be supplied with positive reinforcement and lasting memories that will remind them that eating healthy can be a pleasant experience. If parents are relaxed and cheerful during mealtime, then children will see that behavior as reference point for all future dining experiences.

Eating healthy doesn't have to be dreaded. In fact, every meal can be turned into a celebration. There is no reason to restrict celebrations for holidays and birthdays. Every opportunity for enjoyment should be taken advantage of, and healthy meals can enrich each celebration.

FiT-KiDS...

GETTING KIDS 'HOOKED' ON FITNESS FUN!

SPECIAL AUTHOR'S NOTE

Physical conditioning and endurance levels are different for every child. Therefore, it is advisable to consult a physician prior to beginning any physical activity and nutrition program.

FIT-KIDS ORDER FORM

Please send me the following item(s);
(check applicable box or boxes)

		QTY	PRICE (each)
☐	<u>"FIT-KIDS"... Getting Kids Hooked On Fitness Fun!</u> book		$19.95
☐	"FIT-KIDS" Wall Chart Of Success with stickers		$10.00
☐	"FIT-KIDS" Awards (1 month supply includes 31 stickers, 4 ribbons, and 1 trophy).		$10.00
☐	"I'm Hooked On Fitness Fun!" T-shirt (specify size of child -S/M/L)		$10.00
☐	"FIT-KIDS" Tote Bag		$15.00

Shipping and handling charge		$ 2.00
	sub-total	
NY STATE RESIDENTS MUST ADD 8 1/4% SALES TAX	**sales tax**	
	total	

NAME _____

ADDRESS _____

Please make check payable to;   **ALLURE PUBLISHING**

Mail your order form to;   **ALLURE PUBLISHING**
1470 Old Country Road
Suite 320
Plainview, NY   11803

About The Author

Mandy Laderer created "FIT-KIDS" in 1986. "FIT-KIDS" is a fitness and nutrition program exclusively designed for children. Mandy travels throughout the entire New York Metropolitan area as an advocate for promoting healthy fitness and eating habits for children. She has appeared on a number of radio and television programs as well as the lecture circuit.

Mandy has written articles with the primary focus on fitness for children for several magazines and newspapers.

In addition to working with children, Mandy has been getting adults "hooked on fitness" as a corporate fitness director for a fitness facility located on Long Island, New York for eight years.

If you would like to schedule a lecture, personal appearance, or a "FIT-KID" promotional event with Mandy Laderer, please submit your requests to;

ALLURE PUBLISHING
1470 Old Country Road
Suite 320
Plainview, NY   11803

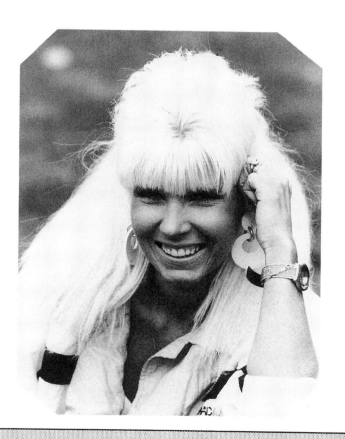